Paleo Diet Recipes 365 Days Of Anti-Inf
By Mercedes Del Rey

DOWNLOAD YOUR FREE PALEO EPIGENETIC DIET EBOOK

AND START LOSING WEIGHT TODAY

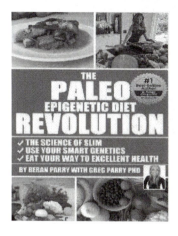

Please search this page over the internet
www.skinnydeliciouslife.com/free-epigenetic-diet-ebook

Paleo Diet Recipes 365 Days Of Anti-Inflammatory Recipes
By Mercedes Del Rey

Paleo Diet Recipes

365 Days

Of

Anti-Inflammatory Recipes

by

Mercedes Del Rey

Paleo Diet Recipes 365 Days Of Anti-Inflammatory Recipes
By Mercedes Del Rey

Copyright © 2017 by Beran Parry

(olw16032017)

All rights reserved. No part of this publication may be reproduced, distributed, or transmitted in any form or by any means, including photocopying, recording, or other electronic or mechanical methods, without the prior written permission of the publisher, except in the case of brief quotations embodied in critical reviews and certain other non-commercial uses permitted by copyright law. For permission requests, write to the publishers' email address: beranparry@gmail.com

Paleo Diet Recipes 365 Days Of Anti-Inflammatory Recipes
By Mercedes Del Rey

SPECIAL FREE GIFT FROM THE PUBLISHER

The PERFECT PALEO RECIPE BUNDLE
4 Life Changing Books
By Beran Parry

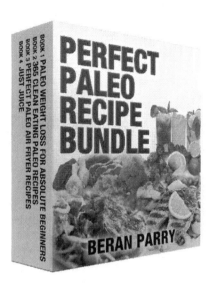

Please search this page over the internet
app.getresponse.com/site2/perfectpaleorecipesbundle?u=mZLi&webforms_id=8541901

Paleo Diet Recipes 365 Days Of Anti-Inflammatory Recipes
By Mercedes Del Rey

FOR MORE BY

MERCEDES DEL REY

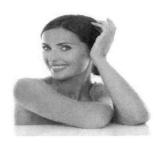

Please search this page over the www.amazon.com
amzn.to/2kSzZnU

Paleo Diet Recipes 365 Days Of Anti-Inflammatory Recipes
By Mercedes Del Rey

INTRODUCTION

Welcome to my world of holistic healing and totally delicious nutrition. My name is Mercedes del Rey but my friends just call me Merche and I am truly fortunate to live in one of the most beautiful places in the world. My home is in the sun-kissed paradise of Andalusia in southern Spain where I am busily planning my holistic wellbeing and nutritional healing centre. This is where I grew up, went to school, studied and graduated before travelling to the US to further my education. My travels and studies have taken me to China and India, Africa and South East Asia and I feel at home wherever I go. I feel I have become what my parents encouraged me to be - a citizen of the world. My purpose in life is to help people to experience the full potential of their wellbeing and I've been guiding and advising individuals on the merits of natural, intelligent nutrition for most of my working life. I want to share my knowledge and experience with you and make a positive difference to the quality of your life

I'm delighted that you have chosen this book full of delicious recipes and hope that you enjoy them all

Paleo Diet Recipes 365 Days Of Anti-Inflammatory Recipes
By Mercedes Del Rey

# Paleo Diet Recipes 365 Days Of Anti-Inflammatory Recipes
By Mercedes Del Rey

Contents

	INTRODUCTION	7
1.	Gutsy Granola	18
2.	Spicy Granola	19
3.	High Protein Breakfast Gold	20
4.	Apple Breakfast Dream	21
5.	Divine Protein Muesli	22
6.	Ultimate Skinny Granola	23
7.	Apple Chia Delight	24
8.	Tasty Apple Almond Coconut Medley	25
9.	Choco Nut Skinny Muesli Balls	26
10.	Sweetie Skinny Crackers	27
11.	Scrambled Eggs with Chilli	28
12.	Basil and Walnut Eggs Divine	29
13.	Spicy Scrambled Eggs	30
14.	Spicy India Omelet	31
15.	Spectacular Spinach Omelet	32
16.	Blushing Blueberry Omelet	33
17.	Mediterranean Supercharger Omelet with Fennel and Dill	34
18.	Outstanding Veggie Omelet	35
19.	Spicy Spinach Bake	36
20.	Delish Veggie Hash With Eggs	37
21.	Spectacular Eggie Salsa	38
22.	Mushrooms, Eggs and Onion Bonanza	39
23.	Avocado and Shrimp Omelet	40
24.	Delish Veggie Breakfast Peppers	41
25.	Breakfast Mexicana	42
26.	Zucchini Casserole	43
27.	Blueberry Nut Casserole	44
28.	Spicy Turkey Stir Fry	45
29.	Turkey and Kale Pasta Casserole	46
30.	Roasted Lemon Herb Chicken	47
31.	Basil Turkey with Roasted Tomatoes	48
32.	Roasted and Filled Tasty Bell Peppers	49
33.	Chili-Garlic Ostrich or Venison Skewers	50
34.	Creamy Chicken Casserole	51
35.	Spectacular Spaghetti and Delish Turkey Balls	52
36.	Sensational Courgette Pasta and Turkey Bolognaise	53
37.	Tempting Turkey Spaghetti Squash Boats	54
38.	Delicious Turkey Veggie Lasagna	55
39.	Ostrich Steak or Venison with Divine Mustard Sauce and Roasted Tomatoes	57
40.	Tantalizing Turkey Pepper Stir-fry	59
41.	Cheeky Chicken Stir Fry	60
42.	Perfect Eastern Turkey Stir-Fry	61

Paleo Diet Recipes 365 Days Of Anti-Inflammatory Recipes
By Mercedes Del Rey

43.	Creamy Curry Stir Fry	62
44.	Sexy Turkey Scramble	63
45.	Turkey Thai Basil	64
46.	Chicken Fennel Stir-Fry	65
47.	Moroccan Madness	66
48.	Thai Baked Fish with Squash Noodles	67
49.	Divine Prawn Mexicana	69
50.	Superior Salmon with Lemon and Thyme OR Use any White fish	70
51.	Spectacular Shrimp Scampi in Spaghetti Sauce	71
52.	Scrumptious Cod in Delish Sauce	72
53.	Delish Baked dill Salmon	73
54.	Prawn garlic Fried "Rice"	74
55.	Lemon and Thyme Super Salmon	75
56.	Delicious Salmon in Herb Crust	76
57.	Salmon Mustard Delish	77
58.	Sexy Spicy Salmon	78
59.	Mouthwatering Stuffed Salmon	79
60.	Spectacular Salmon	80
61.	Creamy Coconut Salmon	81
62.	Salmon Dill Bonanza	82
63.	Sexy Shrimp Cocktail	83
64.	Gambas al Ajillo--Sizzling Garlic Shrimp	84
65.	Garlic Lemon Shrimp Bonanza	85
66.	Courgette Pesto and Shrimp	86
67.	Easy Shrimp Stir Fry	87
68.	Delectable Shrimp Scampi	88
69.	Citrus Shrimp Delux	89
70.	Sexy Garlic Shrimp	90
71.	Shrimp Cakes Delux	91
72.	Shrimp Spinach Spectacular	92
73.	Prawn Salad Boats	93
74.	Cheeky Curry Shrimp	94
75.	Courgette Shrimp Noodles	95
76.	Sexy Shrimp on Sticks	96
77.	Delicious Fish Stir Fry	97
78.	Sexy Shrimp with Delish Veggie Stir Fry	98
79.	Skinny Delicious Slaw	99
80.	Turkey Eastern Surprise	100
81.	Mediterranean Turkey Delish Salad	101
82.	Skinny Delicious Turkey Divine	102
83.	Chicken Basil Avo Salad	103
84.	Skinny Chicken salad	104
85.	Turkey Taco Salad	105
86.	Cheeky Turkey Salad	106

Paleo Diet Recipes 365 Days Of Anti-Inflammatory Recipes
By Mercedes Del Rey

87.	Macadamia Chicken Salad	107
88.	Rosy Chicken Supreme Salad	108
89.	Turkey Sprouts Salad	110
90.	Delicious Chicken Salad	111
91.	Avocado Tuna Salad	112
92.	Classic Tuna Salad	113
93.	Artichoke Tuna Delight	114
94.	Tasty Tuna Stuffed Tomato	115
95.	Advanced Avocado Tuna Salad	116
96.	Sexy Italian Tuna Salad	117
97.	Divine Chicken or Turkey and Baby Bok Choy Salad	118
98.	Mediterranean Medley Salad	119
99.	Spicy Eastern Salad	120
100.	Basil Avocado Bonanza Salad	121
101.	Chinese Divine Salad	122
102.	Divinely Delish Salad Surprise	123
103.	Avocado Salad with Cilantro and Lime	124
104.	Mexican Medley Salad	125
105.	Macadamia Nut Chicken/Turkey Salad	126
106.	Red Cabbage Bonanza Salad	127
107.	Spectacular Sprouts Salad	129
108.	Avocado Egg Salad	130
109.	Avocado Divine Salad	131
110.	Classic Waldorf Salad	132
111.	Artichoke Heart & Turkey Salad Radicchio Cups	133
112.	Tempting Tuna Stuffed Tomato	134
113.	Incredibly Delish Avocado Tuna Salad	135
114.	Italian Tuna Bonanza Salad	136
115.	Asian Aspiration Salad	137
116.	Tasty Carrot Salad	138
117.	Creamy Carrot Salad	139
118.	Vegetarian Curry with Squash	140
119.	Saucy Gratin with Creamy Cauliflower Bonanza	141
120.	Egg Bok Choy and Basil Stir-Fry	142
121.	Skinny Eggie Vegetable Stir Fry	143
122.	Rucola Salad	144
123.	Tasty Spring Salad	145
124.	Spinach and Dandelion Pomegranate Salad	146
125.	Pure Delish Spinach Salad	147
126.	Sexy Salsa Salad	148
127.	Eastern Avo Salad	149
128.	Curry Coconut Salad	150
129.	Jalapeno Salsa	151
130.	Beet Sprout Divine Salad	152

Paleo Diet Recipes 365 Days Of Anti-Inflammatory Recipes
By Mercedes Del Rey

131.	Divine Carrot Salad	153
132.	Cauliflower Couscous	154
133.	Mouthwatering Mushroom Salad	155
134.	Skinny Sweet Potato Salad	156
135.	Fabulous Brownie Treats	157
136.	Rose Banana Delicious Brownies	158
137.	Pristine Pumpkin Divine	159
138.	Secret Brownies	160
139.	Spectacular Spinach Brownies	161
140.	Choco-coco Brownies	162
141.	Coco – Walnut Brownie Bites	163
142.	Best Ever Banana Surprise Cake	164
143.	Choco Cookie Delight	166
144.	Choco Triple Delight	167
145.	Peach and Almond Cake	169
146.	Apple Cinnamon Walnut Bonanza	170
147.	Chestnut- Cacao Cake	171
148.	Extra Dark Choco Delight	172
149.	Nut Butter Truffles	173
150.	Fetching Fudge	174
151.	Choco – Almond Delights	175
152.	Chococups	176
153.	Choco Coco Cookies	177
154.	Apple Spice Spectacular	178
155.	Absolute Almond Bites	179
156.	Eastern Spice Delights	180
157.	Berry Ice Cream and Almond Delight	181
158.	Creamy Caramely Ice Cream	182
159.	Cheeky Cherry Ice	183
160.	Choco - Coconut Berry Ice	184
161.	Creamy Berrie Pie	185
162.	Peachy Creamy Peaches	186
163.	Spiced Apple Bake	187
164.	Sexy Dessert Pan	188
165.	Pretty Pumpkin Delights	190
166.	Macadamia Pineapple Bonanza	192
167.	Lemony Lemon Delights	194
168.	Gorgeous Berry Smoothie	195
169.	Tempting Coconut Berry Smoothie	196
170.	Volumptious Vanilla Hot Drink	197
171.	Almond Butter Smoothies	198
172.	Choco Walnut Delight	199
173.	Raspberry Hemp Smoothie	200
174.	Choco Banana Smoothie	201

Paleo Diet Recipes 365 Days Of Anti-Inflammatory Recipes
By Mercedes Del Rey

175.	Blueberry Almond Smoothie	202
176.	Hazelnut Butter and Banana Smoothie	203
177.	Vanilla Blueberry Smoothie	204
178.	Chocolate Raspberry Smoothie	205
179.	Peach Smoothie	206
180.	Zesty Citrus Smoothie	207
181.	Apple Smoothie	208
182.	Pineapple Smoothie	209
183.	Strawberry Smoothie	210
184.	Pineapple Coconut Deluxe Smoothie	211
185.	Divine Vanilla Smoothie	212
186.	Coco Orange Delish Smoothie	213
187.	Baby Kale Pineapple Smoothie	214
188.	Sumptuous Strawberry Coconut Smoothie	215
189.	Blueberry Bonanza Smoothies	216
190.	Divine Peach Coconut Smoothie	217
191.	Tantalizing Key Lime Pie Smoothie	218
192.	High Protein and Nutritional Delish Smoothie	219
193.	Pineapple Protein Smoothie	220
194.	Raspberry Coconut Smoothie	221
195.	Ginger Carrot Protein Smoothie	222
196.	Delish Banana Nut Muffins	223
197.	Delightful Cinnamon Apple Muffins	224
198.	Healthy Breakfast Bonanza Muffins	225
199.	Perfect Pumpkin Seeds	226
200.	Gorgeous Spicy Nuts	227
201.	Krunchy Yummy Kale Chips	228
202.	Delicious Cinnamon Apple Chips	229
203.	Gummy Citrus Snack	230
204.	Skinny Veggie Dip	231
205.	Divine Butternut Chips	232
206.	Outstanding Orange Skinny Snack	233
207.	Spicy Pumpkin Seed Bonanza	234
208.	Delectable Chocolate-Frosted Doughnuts	235
209.	Eggplant Divine	236
210.	Choco Apple Nachos	237
211.	Skinny Delicious Snack Bars	238
212.	Pumpkin Vanilla Delight	239
213.	Skinny Quicky Crackers	240
214.	Delectable Parsnip Chips	241
215.	Spicy Crunchy Skinny Snack	242
216.	Raw Hemp Kale Bars	243
217.	Skinny Trail Mix	244
218.	Anti-Aging Fruit Delights	245

Paleo Diet Recipes 365 Days Of Anti-Inflammatory Recipes
By Mercedes Del Rey

219.	Paleo Rosemary Sweet Potato Crunches	246
220.	Apple Peach Skinny Bars	247
221.	Spicy Fried Almonds	248
222.	Zucchini Avocado Hummus	249
223.	Skinny Power Snack	250
224.	Skinny Salsa	251
225.	Divine Turkey Stuffed Tomatoes	252
226.	Curried Nutty Delish	253
227.	Skinny Chips	254
228.	Zesty Zucchini Pesto Roll-ups	255
229.	Butternut Squash-raw Veggie Dip	256
230.	Skinny Power Balls	257
231.	Chocolate Goji Skinny Bars	258
232.	Delish Cashew Butter Treats	259
233.	Roasted Tasty Tomato Soup	260
234.	Thai Coconut Turkey Soup	261
235.	Cheeky Chicken Soup	262
236.	Triple Squash Delight Soup	263
237.	Ginger Carrot Delight Soup	264
238.	Wonderful Watercress Soup	265
239.	Curried Butternut Soup	266
240.	Celery Cashew Cream Soup	267
241.	Mighty Andalusian Gazpacho	268
242.	Munchy Mushroom Soup	269
243.	Tempting Tomato Basil Soup	270
244.	Healing Chicken/Turkey Vegetable Soup	271
245.	Sumptuous Saffron Turkey Cauliflower Soup	273
246.	Delicious Masala Soup	274
247.	Creamy Chicken Soup	275
248.	Delicious Lemon-Garlic Soup	276
249.	Turkey Squash Soup	277
250.	Roasted Winter Vegetable Turkey Soup	278
251.	Jam and 'Cream' Cupcakes	279
252.	Delicious Yellow Cupcake Recipe	280
253.	Perfect Pear & Nutmeg Cupcakes	281
254.	Xmas Chocolate Chip Cupcakes	282
255.	Boston Cream Pie Cupcake Bonanza	283
256.	Vanilla Bean Cupcakes with Mocha Buttercream	285
257.	Meaty Meatloaf Cupcakes	286
258.	Gushing Guava Cupcakes with Whipped Guava Frosting	287
259.	Blushing Blueberry Muffin Recipe	289
260.	Healthy Carrot Ginger Muffins	290
261.	Pecan Muffins	291
262.	Temptingly Perfect Plantain Drop	292

Paleo Diet Recipes 365 Days Of Anti-Inflammatory Recipes
By Mercedes Del Rey

263.	Sweety Potato Muffins	293
264.	Zesty Zucchini Muffins	294
265.	Cozy Coconut Flour Muffins	295
266.	Lemon Mousse Mouthwatering Cupcakes	296
267.	Sexy Savory Muffins	297
268.	Molten Lava Chocolate Cupcake	298
269.	Party Carrot Cupcakes	299
270.	Cinnamon Chocolate Chip Muffins	300
271.	Strawberry Shortcake Cupcakes	301
272.	Thin Mint Mini Cupcakes	303
273.	Lemon-Coconut Petit Fours	304
274.	Blushing Blueberry Cupcakes	306
275.	Delicious Morning Cupcakes	307
276.	Cheerful Coffee Cupcake	308
277.	Luscious Lemon Poppy Seed Cupcake	309
278.	Strawberry chia Cupcake	310
279.	Triple Coconut Cupcakes	311
280.	Lemon-Coconut Muffins	312
281.	Chocolate Banana Muffins	313
282.	Delicious English Cupcakes	314
283.	Amazing Almond Flour Cupcakes	315
284.	Delightful Cinnamon Apple Muffins	316
285.	Delish Banana Nut Muffins	317
286.	Apple Cinnamon Muffins	318
287.	Apple Cardamom Cupcakes	319
288.	Chocolate Olive Oil Cupcakes	321
289.	One-Bowl Coconut Flour Cupcakes	323
290.	Meatloaf Cupcakes	324
291.	Gluten Free Banana Nut Bread	325
292.	Pumpkin crepes	326
293.	Red Coconut Smoothie	327
294.	Briana's House Low Carb Chocolate Chip Cookies	328
295.	Coconut Vanilla Surprise	329
296.	Tempting Coconut Berry Smoothie	330
297.	Pineapple Coconut Deluxe Smoothie	331
298.	Sumptuous Strawberry Coconut Smoothie	332
299.	Divine Peach Coconut Smoothie	333
300.	Raspberry Coconut Smoothie	334
301.	Sweet Melon	335
302.	CINNAMON Coconut Surprise	336
303.	Low Carb Fried Zucchini	337
304.	Slow Cooker Paleo Mexican Breakfast Casserole	338
305.	Paleo Pumpkin Pie Smoothie	339
306.	Paleo Cookie Butter	340

Paleo Diet Recipes 365 Days Of Anti-Inflammatory Recipes
By Mercedes Del Rey

307.	Paleo-friendly Coconut Chocolate Coffee Cake	342
308.	Grain Free Steamed Christmas Puddings – GAPS & Paleo Friendly	343
309.	Paleo Antioxidant Berry Shake	344
310.	Perfect Paleo Loaf	345
311.	Raw Pineapple Coconut Vegan Cheesecake	346
312.	Nutritious Paleo Tortillas	347
313.	Perfect Paleo Bananacado Fudge Cupcakes	348
314.	Paleo Sticky Date Pudding Cupcakes	349
315.	Vanilla Paleo Cupcakes	350
316.	Paleo Vanilla Cupcakes	352
317.	Paleo Chocolate Cupcake with "Peanut Butter" Frosting	353
318.	Addictive & Healthy Paleo Nachos	354
319.	Homemade Paleo Tortilla Chips	356
320.	Paleo Chocolate Cookies (I Can't Get Enough of These)	357
321.	Easy Paleo Shepherd's Pie	358
322.	Paleo Apple Pie Cupcakes with Cinnamon Frosting	359
323.	Paleo French Toast with Blueberry Syrup	360
324.	The Best Paleo Brownies (Chocolaty Goodness)	361
325.	Paleo Chocolate Cranberry Muffins	362
326.	Salt and Vinegar Zucchini Chips	363
327.	Nutritious Paleo Tortillas	364
328.	Perfect Paleo Bananacado Fudge Cupcakes	365
329.	Incredibly Easy Paleo Chicken Soup	366
330.	Paleo Chicken Soup	367
331.	Paleo Chicken Soup with Nuddles	368
332.	PALEO CROCK POT CHICKEN SOUP	369
333.	Paleo Stuffed Breakfast Peppers	370
334.	Blushing Beet Salad	371
335.	Cheeky Chicken Salad	372
336.	Melting Mustard Chicken	373
337.	Easy Paleo Spaghetti Squash & Meatballs	374
338.	Paleo Pulled Pork Sliders	375
339.	Basic Balsamic Steak Marinade	376
340.	Lemon Tilapia Ajillo	377
341.	Paleo crock Bone Broth	378
342.	Paleo Phobroth	379
343.	Fantastic Paleo Broth	381
344.	Tasty Tomato Tilapia	382
345.	Beet Sprout Divine Salad	383
346.	Paleo Keto Bone Broth	384
347.	Faux Paleo Napoleon	386
348.	Fish Fillet Delux	387
349.	Roasted Paleo Citrus and Herb Chicken	388
350.	Stove-top "Cheesy" Paleo Chicken Casserole	389

Paleo Diet Recipes 365 Days Of Anti-Inflammatory Recipes
By Mercedes Del Rey

351. Homemade Herbed Paleo Mayonnaise 390
352. Homemade Paleo Ketchup with a Kick 391
353. Homemade Paleo Honey Mustard from Scratch 392
354. All-Natural Homemade Paleo Apple Butter 393
355. Homemade Paleo BBQ Sauce (YUM) 394
356. Basil Pesto 395
357. Paleo Chicken Tortilla Soup 396
358. Paleo Eggs Benedict on Artichoke Hearts 397
359. Hearty Paleo Jambalaya 398
360. Shrimp & Grits (Paleo Style) 399
361. How to Make Paleo Cauliflower "Rice" 400
362. Paleo Cocoa Puffs 401
363. Tantalizing Prawn Skewers 402
364. Paleo BLT Frittata 403
365. Extra Easy Broth 404

Paleo Diet Recipes 365 Days Of Anti-Inflammatory Recipes
By Mercedes Del Rey

1. Gutsy Granola

Ingredients:
1 cup cashews
3/4 cup almonds
1/4 cup pumpkin seeds, shelled
1/4 cup sunflower seeds, shelled
1/2 cup unsweetened coconut flakes
1/4 cup coconut oil
Stevia to taste
1 tsp vanilla
low sodium salt to taste

Instructions:
Preheat oven to 300 degrees F. Line a baking sheet with parchment paper. Place the cashews, almonds, coconut flakes and pumpkin seeds into a blender and pulse to break the mixture into smaller pieces.

In a large microwave-safe bowl, melt the coconut oil, vanilla, and stevia together for 40-50 seconds. Add in the mixture from the blender and the sunflower seeds, and stir to coat.

Spread the mixture out onto the baking sheet and cook for 20-25 minutes, stirring once, until the mixture is lightly browned. Remove from heat. Add low sodium salt.

Press the granola mixture together to form a flat, even surface. Cool for about 15 minutes, and then break into pieces.

2. Spicy Granola

Ingredients:
1 ½ cups almond flour
1/3 cup coconut oil
2 tsp cinnamon
2 tsp nutmeg
2 tsp vanilla extract
½ cup walnuts
½ cup coconut flakes
¼ cup hemp seeds
low sodium salt, to taste

Instructions:
Preheat oven to 275 degrees Fahrenheit.

Combine all ingredients in a large mixing bowl and mix well... melt down the coconut oil a little bit before adding it

Spread mixture into one flat layer on a greased baking sheet.

Bake for 40-50 minutes, or until mixture is toasted to your liking.

Remove from oven and allow to cool before serving, then transfer into a plastic container.

3. High Protein Breakfast Gold

Ingredients:
1/2 cup (c). Flax-Meal, golden
1/2 c. Chia seed
Stevia liquid to taste
2 tbs. dark ground cinnamon
1 tbs. hemp protein powder
2 tbs. coconut oil, melted
1 tsp. vanilla extract
3/4 c. + 2 tbs. hot water

Instructions:
Begin to spread the dough out until its super thin, onto a parchment paper lined cookie sheet. Bake at 325 for 15 minutes, then drop it down to 300 and leave for 30 minutes.

Before dropping it, pull out the sheet and cut it. Put it back into the oven exactly like this, don't separate the pieces.

When the 30 minutes are up, pull it out and separate the pieces. Drop the pieces to 200 degrees F for 1 hour. They will be completely dried out at this point. Enjoy with almond or other nut milk!

4. Apple Breakfast Dream

Ingredients:
2 Cup (C) raw walnuts
1 C raw macadamia nuts
2 apples, peeled and diced
1 Tbsp coconut oil
1 Tbsp ground cinnamon
2 C almond milk
1 14 oz can full fat coconut milk

Instructions:
Combine nuts and dates in a food processor until ground into a fine meal, about 1 minute; set aside.

Saute apples over medium heat in coconut oil until lightly browned, about 5 minutes.

Add nut mixture and cinnamon to apples and stir to incorporate, about 1 minute.

Reduce heat to low and add coconut and almond milk.

Stirring occasionally, let mixture cook uncovered until thickened, about 25 minutes.

5. Divine Protein Muesli

Ingredients:
1 cup unsweetened unsulfured coconut flakes
1 tbsp chopped walnuts\
1 tbsp raw almonds (~10)
1 tbsp chocolate chips (dark and sugar free)
1/2 tsp cinnamon
1 cup unsweetened almond milk
1 scoop hemp protein

Instructions:
In a medium bowl layer coconut flakes, walnuts, almonds and chocolate chips.

Sprinkle with cinnamon.

Pour cold almond milk over the muesli and eat with a spoon.

6. Ultimate Skinny Granola

Ingredients:
1 cup of unsweetened coconut milk or unsweetened almond milk
Stevia liquid to taste
1 tablespoon each of unsalted …
pecan pieces
walnut pieces
almonds
pistachios
raw pine nuts
raw sunflower/safflower seeds
raw pumpkin seeds
2 Tablespoons of frozen or fresh berry selection (e.g. blueberries, blackberries, raspberries, strawberries, or other kinds etc)

Instructions:
Put all the nuts & seeds in a breakfast bowl.

add a teaspoon of pure liquid stevia and stir it well in.

Add the berries and milk.

If using frozen berries, wait for 2-3 minutes for them to get warmer.

The berries will now release some color into the milk, making it look really interesting. Enjoy!

7. Apple Chia Delight

Ingredients:
2c organic chia seeds (black or white)
1c organic hemp hearts
1/2 chopped fresh apple
2tbsp real cinnamon
1 tsp low sodium salt
optional: 1/2c chopped nuts of your choice

Instructions:
Throw all of this together, mix it up, and enjoy with almond milk. Stevia to taste.

8. Tasty Apple Almond Coconut Medley

Ingredients:
one-half apple cored and roughly diced
handful of sliced almonds
handful of unsweetened coconut
generous dose of cinnamon
1 pinch of low sodium salt

Instructions:
Pulse in the food processor to desired consistency–smaller is better for the little ones! Serve with almond milk, or creamy coconut milk.

9. Choco Nut Skinny Muesli Balls

Ingredients:
1 cup of raw almonds
1 Tablespoon of coconut oil
¼ teaspoon low sodium salt
2 Tablespoon Coconut flour
1 egg white
2 Tablespoon plus 1 teaspoon of Cacao powder
pure liquid stevia to taste

Instructions:

First grind the almonds in a food processor or blender until you have a flour.

Add the ground almonds, low sodium salt, coconut flour, egg white, pure liquid stevia and cacao power to a bowl and mix with a spoon until you have a dough.

Either:

a) Place the dough onto a piece of parchment paper. Place a second piece of parchment paper over the top and roll it until it is ¼" thick. With a wet knife, score it into 1" squares. Place the parchment paper on a baking sheet when finished.

Or

b) Take a small pinch of the dough and roll into a ¼ round ball and set on a baking sheet lined with parchment paper.

Turn on your oven and set to 350 degrees and bake for 15 - 18 minutes for cereal balls or bake for 8 to 12 minutes for flat cereal.

Remove from the oven and let cool on the pan.

Top with your favorite nut or seed milk and enjoy!

10. Sweetie Skinny Crackers

Ingredients:
1 egg
pure liquid stevia to taste
1 Tbspn coconut oil, melted
1.5 cups almond flour
5 cup coconut flour
1 teaspoon cinnamon

Instructions:
Preheat oven to 350°

In a large bowl, whisk together the egg, pure liquid stevia and melted coconut oil

Add the coconut and almond flour and stir to combine.

Give the dough a couple of kneads so it's well incorporated.

Turn the dough onto a piece of parchment paper and flatten a bit with your hands.

Place another piece of parchment on top and roll out with a rolling pin until it's about 1/8 inch thick.

Remove the top piece of parchment and cut the dough into 1/4 inch squares for cereal, and about 2"x3" for crackers

Sprinkle the cinnamon into the dough mixture.

Slide the dough with the bottom parchment paper onto a baking sheet and bake for 15 minutes.

Turn down the oven to 325° and bake for another 10-15 minutes, or until the cereal / crackers are crisp.

11. Scrambled Eggs with Chilli

Ingredients:
4 fresh green chillies with skins removed
2 tablespoons (30g or 1 oz) coconut oil
1 small onion, peeled and finely chopped
6 eggs
1/4 cup (62ml or 2 fl oz) coconut milk
low sodium salt to taste

Instructions:
After removing chilli skins, remove and discard seeds and finely chop remaining chilli.

Beat eggs, coconut milk and salt in a bowl and set aside.

Heat oil in a medium size saucepan over a medium heat.

Reduce heat to low and add egg mixture to saucepan and mix well.

Scatter chilies over mixture.

Cook over a low heat until eggs are cooked.

Serves 4. Serve hot.

12. Basil and Walnut Eggs Divine

Ingredients:
3 organic eggs
1/2 cup fresh basil, chopped
1/3 cup walnuts, chopped
salt and pepper

Instructions:
Whisk eggs in a bowl then place in a frying pan on medium heat, stirring constantly.

When the eggs are almost cooked, add the basil and continue cooking for a further 1 minute or until eggs are fully cooked.

Add salt and pepper to taste.

Remove from heat and stir in the walnuts before serving.

13. Spicy Scrambled Eggs

Ingredients:
1 tablespoon extra virgin olive oil
1 red onion, finely chopped
1 medium green pepper, cored, seeded, and finely chopped
1 chilli, seeded and cut into thin strips
3 ripe tomatoes, peeled, seeded, and chopped
Salt and freshly ground black pepper
4 large organic eggs

Instructions:

Heat the olive oil in a large, heavy, preferably nonstick skillet over medium heat.

Add the onion and cook until soft, 6 to 7 minutes.

Add the pepper and chilli and continue cooking until soft, another 4 to 5 minutes.

Add in the tomatoes, and salt and pepper to taste and cook uncovered, over low heat for 10 minutes.

Add the eggs, stirring them into the mixture to distribute.

Cover the skillet and cook until the eggs are set but still fluffy and tender, about 7 to 8 minutes. Divide between 4 plates and serve.

14. Spicy India Omelet

Ingredients:
3 Eggs
1 Onion, chopped
4 Green Chilli (optional)
1/4 cup Coconut grated
Low sodium Salt as required
1 tblspoon olive oil

Instructions:
Beat the Eggs severely.

Mix chopped onion, rounded green chilli, salt and grated coconuts with eggs.

Heat oil on a medium-low heat, in a pan.

Pour the mixture in the form of pancakes and cook it on the both sides.

15. Spectacular Spinach Omelet

Ingredients:
2 eggs
1.5 cups raw spinach
coconut oil, about 1 tbsp
1/3 c tomatoes and onion salsa (lightly fried in pan)
1 tbsp fresh cilantro

Instructions:
Melt coconut oil on medium in frying pan. Add spinach, cook until mostly wilted. Beat eggs and add to pan.

Flip once the egg sets around the edge. When it's almost done add the salsa on top just to warm it. Move to plate and add cilantro. Serves one.

16. Blushing Blueberry Omelet

Ingredients:
2 eggs
1 tsp. vanilla extract
coconut oil
1/2 c. blueberries
Stevia to taste

Instructions:
Lightly beat two eggs and vanilla extract in a bowl. Heat 6" non-stick pan over medium heat.

While pan is heating, heat half the blueberries in a saucepan until juices flow.

Add coconut oil to non-stick pan and coat evenly.

When thoroughly heated, add egg mixture. Turn once and let sit.

When eggs are about 70% settled, turn again. There should be a nice crispy layer around the side of the pan.

When it starts to separate from the side, add fresh and cooked blueberries to omelet, reserving a few for garnish.

Crispy layer should really be pulling away from pan now.

Use a fork to help fold the omelet over. Slide on to plate, top with reserved blueberry filling, and enjoy!

17. Mediterranean Supercharger Omelet with Fennel and Dill

Ingredients:
2 tablespoons olive oil, divided
2 cups thinly sliced fresh fennel bulb, fronds chopped and reserved
8 cherry tomatoes
5 large eggs, beaten to blend with 1/4 teaspoon salt and 1/4 teaspoon ground black pepper
1 1/2 tablespoons chopped fresh dill

Instructions:
Add remaining 1 tablespoon oil to same skillet; heat over medium-high heat.

Add beaten eggs and cook until eggs are just set in center, tilting skillet and lifting edges of omelet with spatula to let uncooked portion flow underneath, about 3 minutes.

Top with fennel mixture. Sprinkle dill over.

Using spatula, fold uncovered half of omelet over; slide onto plate.

Garnish with chopped fennel and serve.

18. Outstanding Veggie Omelet

Ingredients:
3 eggs, beaten
1 carrot, matchstick cut
3 scallions, diagonal sliced
1 handful tiny broccoli florets or whatever leftover veggies you have
Bits of leftover cooked turkey
Safflower oil
Low sodium salt

Instructions:
Heat oil in a wok or large cast iron skillet over medium heat, until hot enough to sizzle a drop of water.

Add broccoli and carrots, stir fry 2 min. until soft.

Add cooked turkey, stir fry 1 min. until heated through. Add scallions and eggs, scramble. Add salt to taste. Serve.

19. Spicy Spinach Bake

Ingredients:
6 eggs
1 bunch fresh spinach chopped (a box of frozen will do if you do not have fresh)
1/2 tsp hot pepper flakes
Olive oil
Low sodium Salt and pepper

Instructions:
Scramble the eggs in a bowl. Add the spinach, low sodium salt and pepper.

Scramble together. Heat a large non-stick skillet with about 1/2 cup olive oil.

When the oil is hot put the hot pepper flakes in then pour the mixture in. When it starts to cook on the bottom, flip it over

Take it out when it is medium scrambled. Let cool and eat.

20. Delish Veggie Hash With Eggs

Ingredients:
2 tablespoon extra virgin olive oil
2 garlic cloves, minced
1/4 cup sweet white onion, chopped
1 cup yellow squash, chopped
1/2 cup mushroom, sliced
Low sodium salt and pepper
1 cup cherry tomatoes, halved
1 cup fresh spinach, chopped
4 eggs, poached or cooked any style
You can substitute the squash with whatever vegetables you have

Instructions:

Heat large non-stick skillet over medium heat. Add olive oil to pan.

Add garlic and onion and saute for 2 minutes, then add chopped squash or your favorite vegetable, cook for 2 more minutes, then add mushrooms. Cook for 5-minutes or until almost compete.

At this point add low sodium salt and pepper, then add tomatoes and spinach and cook until spinach wilts. Drain well before plating.

While finishing this prepare eggs to your liking in another pan.

To serve, drained hash mixture to and then add to individual plates. On top of hash add 2 cooked eggs per person.

21. Spectacular Eggie Salsa

Ingredients:
2 pounds fresh ripe tomatoes, peeled and coarsely chopped
2 to 3 serrano or jalapeño chiles, seeded for a milder sauce, and chopped
2 garlic cloves, peeled, halved, green shoots removed
1/2 small onion, chopped
2 tablespoons oil
Low sodium salt to taste
4 to 8 eggs (to taste)
Chopped cilantro for garnish

Instructions:
Place the tomatoes, chiles, garlic and onion in a blender and puree, retaining a bit of texture.

Heat 1 tablespoon of the oil over high heat in a large, heavy nonstick skillet, until a drop of puree will sizzle when it hits the pan.

Add the puree and cook, stirring, for four to ten minutes, until the sauce thickens, darkens and leaves a trough when you run a spoon down the middle of the pan. It should just begin to stick to the pan.

Season to taste with salt, and remove from the heat. Keep warm while you fry the eggs.

Warm four plates. Fry the eggs in a heavy skillet over medium-high heat.

Use the remaining tablespoon of oil if necessary. Cook them sunny side up, until the whites are solid but the yolks still runny.

Season with salt and pepper, and turn off the heat. Place one or two fried eggs on each plate.

Spoon the hot salsa over the whites of the eggs, leaving the yolks exposed if possible. Sprinkle with cilantro and serve.

22. Mushrooms, Eggs and Onion Bonanza

Ingredients:
1 medium onion, finely diced
1/4 cup coconut oil
10-12 medium white mushrooms, finely chopped
12 hard boiled eggs, peeled and finely chopped
Freshly ground black pepper to taste

Instructions:
Saute the onion in coconut oil until golden brown.

Add the mushrooms and saute another 5 minutes or so, stirring frequently, until mushrooms are softened and turned dark.

Remove from heat and let cool.

Mix together with the eggs and pepper. Chill until ready to serve.

23. Avocado and Shrimp Omelet

Ingredients:
6 eggs
2 Tbsp. chopped parsley
2 Tbsp. lemon juice, divided
1/4 tsp. salt
1/8 tsp. cayenne pepper
1 large* ripe avocado, diced
1 1/2 Tbsp. avocado oil
3 oz. bay shrimp
3 parsley sprigs

Instructions:
Beat together eggs, parsley, 3/4 of the lemon juice, salt, and cayenne pepper; reserve.

Gently toss avocado with remaining lemon juice; reserve.

Heat oil in an omelet pan. (Use a large omelet pan for four or more servings.)

Pour egg mixture into pan.

Cook over medium heat, lifting edges and tilting pan to allow uncooked egg to run under, until set but still moist on top.

Scatter reserved avocado and shrimp over omelet.

Fold omelet in half; heat another minute or two.

Slide onto a warmed serving plate; garnish with parsley sprigs.

To serve, cut omelet into wedges.

24. Delish Veggie Breakfast Peppers

Ingredients:
2 bell peppers – your choice of color
4 eggs
1 cup white mushrooms
1 cup broccoli
¼ tsp cayenne pepper
low sodium salt and pepper, to taste

Instructions:
Preheat oven to 375 degrees Fahrenheit.

Dice up your vegetables of choice.

In a medium sized bowl, mix eggs, low sodium salt, pepper, cayenne pepper, and vegetables.

Cut peppers into equal halves. A tip:

Core the peppers so that they're clean enough to add the filling.

Pour a quarter of the egg / vegetable mix into each pepper halve, adding more vegetables to the top to fill in any empty space.

Place on baking sheet and cook approximately 35 minutes.

25. Breakfast Mexicana

Ingredients:
For the tortillas:
2 eggs
2 egg whites
1/2 cup water
4 tsp ground flaxseed
Pinch of low sodium salt

For the filling:
1 avocado, diced
1/4 cup red bell pepper, finely diced
1/4 cup onion, finely diced
1/4 cup baked cod or other protein
Handful of spinach leaves
1 tsp coconut oil

Instructions:
In a small bowl, whisk together the ingredients for the tortilla. Preheat the oven

Heat a 10-inch non-stick skillet over medium heat and coat well with coconut oil spray.

Pour half of the tortilla mixture into the pan and swirl to evenly distribute.

Using a metal spatula, loosen the edges of the tortilla from the pan.

Cook a couple of minutes until golden brown on the bottom, and then carefully slide the spatula under the tortilla to loosen it from the bottom of the pan. Do not flip yet.

Place the pan under the broiler for 3-4 minutes until the tortilla gets a little bubbly.

Remove the tortilla from the pan, setting on a piece of aluminum foil. Repeat with other half of tortilla mixture.

After the tortillas are done broiling, preheat the oven to 400 degrees F. In a separate small pan, heat the coconut oil over medium heat.

Add the onions and peppers and sauté for 5-8 minutes, until soft. Add the spinach into the pan and wilt.

Place all of the fillings down the center of the tortillas and wrap tightly. Place into the oven for 5-8 minutes to set. It's so delish!

26. Zucchini Casserole

Ingredients:
3 large zucchini
1/2 red onion, chopped
1/2 cup mushrooms
5 eggs
1 tsp low sodium salt
Freshly ground black pepper, to taste

Instructions:
Preheat oven to 375 degrees F..

Grate all of the zucchini and put into a large bowl.

In a separate bowl, beat the eggs with low sodium salt and pepper.

Combine all of the ingredients, in the large bowl and mix together. You want to have enough eggs to coat the whole mixture.

Warm about a 1/2 tablespoon of olive oil in the skillet over medium heat.

Add the zucchini mixture into the pan. Cover and cook about 5 minutes until the eggs start to set on the bottom.

Transfer to the oven and bake for 12-15 minutes, until the eggs are firm. Remove and let rest for 5-10 minutes, then serve.

27. Blueberry Nut Casserole

Ingredients:
Crush one cup almonds, walnuts and pecans with one teaspoon olive oil and bake in the oven at 200 for 20 minutes
2 cups frozen blueberries
5 eggs
1 cup almond milk
Stevia to taste
1 tsp vanilla extract
1 tsp cinnamon
Pinch of nutmeg

Instructions:
Preheat the oven to 350 degrees F. Grease an 8x8-inch baking dish with coconut oil spray. Place the nut crust and blueberries into the dish.

Whisk together the eggs, almond milk, stevia, vanilla, and cinnamon in a medium bowl.

Pour the egg mixture over the crust and blueberries. Lightly stir to coat.

Bake for 35-45 minutes. Remove from the oven and allow the casserole to rest for 15 minutes before serving.

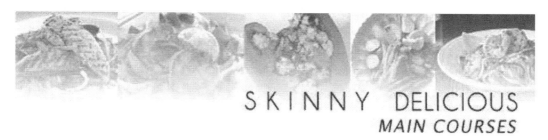

SKINNY DELICIOUS
MAIN COURSES

28. Spicy Turkey Stir Fry

Ingredients:
2 lbs. boneless skinless chicken or turkey breasts, cut into 1-inch slices
2 tbsp coconut oil
1 tsp cumin seeds
1/2 each green, red, and orange bell pepper, thinly sliced
1 tsp garam masala
2 tsp freshly ground pepper
low sodium salt, to taste
Scallions, for garnish

For the marinade:
1/2 cup coconut cream
1 clove garlic, minced
1 tsp ginger, minced
1 tbsp freshly ground pepper
2 tsp low sodium salt
1/4 tsp turmeric

Instructions:
Place all of the marinade ingredients into a Ziploc bag. Add the chicken, close the bag, and shake to coat.

Marinate in the refrigerator for at least 30 minutes, or up to 6 hours.

In a wok or large sauté pan, melt the coconut oil over medium-high heat. Add the cumin seeds and cook for 2-3 minutes.

Add the marinated chicken and let cook for 5 minutes. Stir the chicken until it begins to brown, and then add the peppers, garam masala, and freshly ground pepper.

Sprinkle with low sodium salt. Cook for 4-5 minutes, stirring regularly, or until the bell pepper is cooked to desired doneness. Serve hot.

29. Turkey and Kale Pasta Casserole

Ingredients:
1 lb. Turkey breast
1 medium spaghetti squash, halved and seeded
Extra virgin olive oil, for drizzling
1 large bunch of kale, de-stemmed, and chopped
1/2 red onion, sliced thin
1/3 cup chicken broth
1/2 cup coconut milk
1 clove garlic, minced
2 tsp Italian seasoning – salt free
low sodium salt and freshly ground pepper, to taste

Instructions:
Preheat the oven to 400 degrees F. Place the squash in the microwave for 3-4 minutes to soften.

Using a sharp knife, cut the squash in half lengthwise. Scoop out the seeds and discard. Place the halves, with the cut side up, on a rimmed baking sheet.

Drizzle with olive oil and sprinkle with low sodium salt and pepper. Roast in the oven for 45-50 minutes, until you can poke the squash easily with a fork.

Let it cool until you can handle it safely. Then scrape the insides with a fork to shred the squash into strands.

Meanwhile, melt the coconut oil in a large oven-safe skillet over medium heat.

Add the turkey breast and brown. Once cooked through, remove to a plate. In the same skillet, add the onion and sauté for 3-4 minutes.

Next add the garlic, Italian seasoning, and kale and cook for 2-3 minutes to slightly wilt the kale.

Pour in the chicken broth and coconut milk and simmer for an additional 2-3 minutes. Remove from heat.

Stir in the cooked turkey. Add the spaghetti squash into the skillet and stir well to combine.

Bake for 15-18 minutes, until the top has slightly browned. Serve hot.

30. Roasted Lemon Herb Chicken

Ingredients:
12 total pieces bone-in chicken thighs and legs
1 medium onion, thinly sliced
1 tbsp dried rosemary
1 tsp dried thyme
1 lemon, sliced thin
1 orange, sliced thin

For the marinade:
5 tbsp extra virgin olive oil
6 cloves garlic, minced
Stevia to taste
Juice of 1 lemon
Juice of 1 orange
1 tbsp Italian seasoning – salt free
1 tsp onion powder
Dash of red pepper flakes
low sodium salt and freshly ground pepper, to taste

Instructions:

Whisk together all of the marinade ingredients in a small bowl. Place the chicken in a baking dish (or a large Ziploc bag) and pour the marinade over it. Marinate for 3 hours to overnight.

Preheat the oven to 400 degrees F. Place the chicken in a baking dish and arrange with the onion, orange, and lemon slices.

Sprinkle with thyme, rosemary, low sodium salt and pepper. Cover with aluminum foil and bake for 30 minutes.

Remove the foil, baste the chicken, and bake for another 30 minutes uncovered, until the chicken is cooked through.

31. Basil Turkey with Roasted Tomatoes

Ingredients:
2 turkey breasts
1 cup mushrooms, chopped
1/2 medium onion, chopped
1-2 tbsp extra virgin olive oil
Half cup thinly sliced fresh basil
low sodium salt and pepper, to taste
1 pint cherry tomatoes
Stevia to taste
Fresh parsley, for garnish

Instructions:
Preheat the oven to 400 degrees F. Place the tomatoes on a baking sheet and drizzle with olive oil and stevia. Sprinkle with low sodium salt and pepper and toss to coat evenly. Bake for 15-20 minutes until soft.

While the tomatoes are roasting, heat one tablespoon of olive oil in a large pan over low heat. Add the onions and mushrooms and cook for 10-12 minutes to soften and caramelize, stirring regularly. Clear a space for the chicken.

Season the turkey with low sodium salt and pepper and then place it in the pan. Simmer for 15 minutes or until the chicken is cooked through. Every 5 minutes or so, spoon the sauce in the pan over the turkey.

To assemble, divide the tomatoes between two plates. Place one turkey breast on each and then spoon the onions, mushrooms, and pan drippings over the turkey. Garnish with parsley.

32. Roasted and Filled Tasty Bell Peppers

Ingredients:
5 large bell peppers
1 tbsp coconut oil
1/2 large onion, diced
1 tsp dried oregano
1/2 tsp low sodium salt
1 lb. ground turkey
1 large zucchini, halved and diced
3 tbsp tomato paste
Freshly ground black pepper, to taste
Fresh parsley, for serving

Instructions:
Preheat the oven to 350 degrees F. Coat a small baking dish with coconut oil spray. Bring a large pot of water to a boil. Cut the stems and very top of the peppers off, removing the seeds. Place in boiling water for 4-5 minutes. Remove from the water and drain face-down on a paper towel.

Heat the coconut oil in a large nonstick pan over medium heat. Add in the onion. Sauté for 3-4 minutes until the onion begins to soften. Stir in the ground turkey, oregano, low sodium salt, and pepper and cook until turkey is browned.

Add the zucchini to the skillet as the turkey finishes cooking. Cook everything together until the zucchini is soft, and then drain any juices from the pan.

Remove the pan from heat and stir in the tomato paste. Bake for 15 minutes.

33. Chili-Garlic Ostrich or Venison Skewers

Ingredients:
6 Wooden Skewers, soaked in cold water for 30 minutes
2 Ostrich or Venison, diced
1 tbsp. Olive Oil
1 tsp. Red Chilies, seeds removed & finely chopped
4 Garlic Cloves, minced
6 tbsp. fresh lemon juice

Instructions:
Preheat oven to 350 F or preheat barbeque grill on high heat.

To make sauce, combine the oil, chilies, garlic, and lemon juice in a small bowl. Set aside for a few minutes.

Thread diced meat onto skewers and place on an oven tray lined with baking paper.

Pour chili and garlic sauce over the chicken, coating well.

Bake in the oven for 30-40 minutes or until chicken is cooked. If cooking on a grill, cook meat or poultry for 5-6 minutes on each side.

Eat with any of the delicious salad recipes.

34. Creamy Chicken Casserole

Ingredients:
2 cups cubed cooked chicken
1 1/2 cups cooked butternut squash
1/2 cup coconut cream,
1/4 cup coconut oil, melted
1 heaping cup green peas, fresh or frozen
1 tbsp apple cider vinegar
1/2 tsp low sodium salt
1/2 tsp oregano
1/2 tsp thyme
1 tbsp fresh parsley

Instructions:
In a large bowl, mash the butternut squash. Stir in the coconut cream, oil, vinegar, low sodium salt, oregano, and thyme.

Once everything is combined, add in chicken and peas.

Place the mixture into a large saucepan and cook over medium heat for 5-8 minutes.

Top with fresh parsley and serve warm.

35. Spectacular Spaghetti and Delish Turkey Balls

Ingredients:
1 spaghetti squash
Extra virgin olive oil,
low sodium salt and pepper
1 tsp dried or fresh oregano

For the sauce:
1 lb ground turkey
1 small onion, chopped
4 cloves garlic, minced
1 tbsp coconut oil
1 tomato, chopped
1/2 jar of tomato sauce
1 tbsp Italian seasoning
low sodium salt and pepper to taste
Fresh basil

Instructions:

Preheat oven to 400 degrees F. Using a sharp knife, cut the squash in half lengthwise. Scoop out the seeds and discard.

Place the halves with the cut side up on a rimmed baking sheet. Drizzle with olive oil and season with low sodium salt, pepper, and oregano. Roast the squash in the oven for 40-45 minutes, until you can poke the squash easily with a fork.

Let it cool until you can handle it safely. Then scrape the insides with a fork to shred the squash into strands.

While the spaghetti squash is roasting, melt coconut oil in a large skillet over medium heat.

Add chopped onion and garlic and cook for 4-5 minutes. Add ground turkey and brown the meat, stirring occasionally. Season with low sodium salt and pepper.

Add the chopped tomato, tomato sauce, and Italian seasoning and stir to combine. Simmer on low heat, stirring occasionally, while the spaghetti squash finishes roasting. Serve over spaghetti squash with basil for garnish.

36. Sensational Courgette Pasta and Turkey Bolognaise

Ingredients:
4 medium zucchini

For the sauce:
1 lb ground turkey
1 small onion, chopped
4 cloves garlic, minced
1 tbsp coconut oil
1 tomato, chopped
1/2 jar of tomato sauce
1 tbsp Italian seasoning
low sodium salt and pepper to taste
Fresh basil, for garnish

Instructions:

Use a julienne peeler to slice the zucchini into noodles, stopping when you reach the seeds. Set aside.

If cooking zucchini noodles, simply add to a skillet and sauté over medium heat for 4-5 minutes.

Melt coconut oil in a large skillet over medium heat. Add chopped onion and garlic and cook for 4-5 minutes.

Add ground turkey and brown the meat, stirring occasionally. Season with low sodium salt and pepper.

Add the chopped tomato, tomato sauce, and Italian seasoning and stir to combine. Simmer on low heat, stirring occasionally.

Add the sauce to the noodles and ENJOY.

37. Tempting Turkey Spaghetti Squash Boats

Ingredients:
1 medium spaghetti squash or 2 small spaghetti squash
1 1/2 lbs. Turkey mashed
1 yellow onion, diced
4 cloves garlic, minced
1 bunch kale
3 tbsp extra virgin olive oil, plus more for drizzling
low sodium salt and pepper
2 tbsp pine nuts, roasted
2 tbsp fresh parsley, chopped

Instructions:

Preheat the oven to 400 degrees F. Place squash in the microwave for 3-4 minutes to soften. Using a sharp knife cut the squash in half lengthwise. Scoop out the seeds and discard.

Place the halves, with the cut side up, on a rimmed baking sheet. Drizzle with olive oil and sprinkle with low sodium salt and pepper.

Roast in the oven for 45-50 minutes, until you can poke the squash easily with a fork. Let cool until you can handle it safely.

Meanwhile, prepare the kale by removing the center stems and either tearing or cutting up the leaves. Heat the olive oil in a large skillet over medium heat.

Add the onion and garlic and sauté for 4-5 minutes. Add the turkey. Cook for 10-12 minutes, stirring regularly, until the turkey is browned and cooked through.

Add the kale and stir. Cook for a few minutes more to wilt the kale. Remove from heat and set aside.

Once cooled, scrape the insides of the spaghetti squash with a fork to shred the squash into strands. Transfer the strands into the skillet with the turkey and toss to combine.

Season to taste with low sodium salt and pepper. Divide the mixture among the squash shells, and then top with pine nuts and parsley to serve.

38. Delicious Turkey Veggie Lasagna

Ingredients:
For the meat sauce:
1 large yellow onion, coarsely chopped
2 cloves garlic, coarsely chopped
2 tbsp extra virgin olive oil
1 1/2 lbs. ground turkey
1/2 cup tomato paste
1/2 cup tomato sauce
1 cup red wine
1 bay leaf
3 sprigs thyme
low sodium salt and freshly ground pepper, to taste

For the lasagna:
1 eggplant, sliced lengthwise thinly
1 tsp low sodium salt
1 tbsp extra virgin olive oil
2 yellow squash, sliced thinly
1/2 cup torn fresh basil leaves
8 oz. white mushrooms, sliced
2 cups fresh spinach
2 large zucchini, sliced lengthwise into ribbons

For the topping:
1/2 head cauliflower
1 tbsp olive oil
1/2 tsp garlic powder
1/2 tsp low sodium salt
Freshly ground pepper, to taste

Instructions:
To make the meat sauce, place the onion and garlic in a food processor and pulse to finely chop.

Heat the olive oil in a heavy-bottomed saucepan over medium heat. Add the onion and garlic and season with low sodium salt and pepper. Cook for 12-15 minutes until beginning to brown, stirring frequently.

Add the turkey to the pot and season with low sodium salt and pepper.

Cook for 15 minutes until browned. Stir in the tomato paste and cook for 2-3 minutes. Add the red wine to the pan and cook for 5 more minutes.

Add the tomato sauce, bay leaf, and thyme to the pan. Bring to a simmer, and then add 1/2 cup water.

Cook at a low simmer for 1 hour, stirring occasionally and adding more water if necessary. Adjust seasonings to taste. Discard the bay leaf and thyme.

Preheat the oven to 350 degrees F. Sprinkle the eggplant with low sodium salt and set aside for 15 minutes to drain. Rinse and pat dry.

Heat one tablespoon of olive oil in a skillet over medium heat. Cook the eggplant for 2-3 minutes per side until golden.

Layer the lasagna in a baking dish. Start by layering the yellow squash as the base. Add one third of the meat sauce on top of that, then lay the eggplant slices, fresh basil, and mushrooms.

Next add the rest of the meat sauce, then the spinach, zucchini, and finally drizzle with olive oil and sprinkle with low sodium salt and pepper. Bake for 40-45 minutes.

While the lasagna is baking, place the cauliflower in a blender and process until it reaches a rice-like consistency.

Add to a skillet and sauté with the olive oil, garlic powder, low sodium salt, and pepper over medium heat.

Cook for 6-8 minutes until soft, adding a tablespoon of water if necessary. After the lasagna has cooked for 20 minutes, sprinkle with the cauliflower and return to the oven for the remaining cooking time. Serve hot.

39. Ostrich Steak or Venison with Divine Mustard Sauce and Roasted Tomatoes

Ingredients:

For the tomatoes:
2 pints cherry tomatoes, halved
2 tbsp extra virgin olive oil
Stevia to taste
low sodium salt and freshly ground pepper

For the cauliflower rice:
1/2 head of cauliflower, chopped coarsely
1/2 small onion, finely diced
1 tbsp coconut oil
1 tbsp fresh parsley, chopped
low sodium salt and freshly ground pepper, to taste

For the meat:
4 Ostrich or venison steaks
Extra virgin olive oil
low sodium salt and freshly ground pepper
Coconut oil, for the pan

For the sauce:
1/4 cup red onion, finely diced
1/4 cup apple cider vinegar
1 cup low sodium chicken stock
1 tbsp whole grain mustard
low sodium salt and freshly ground pepper, to taste

Instructions:

Preheat the oven to 400 degrees F. Place the tomatoes on a baking sheet and drizzle with olive oil and honey. Sprinkle with low sodium salt and pepper and toss to coat evenly. Bake for 15-20 minutes until soft.

While the tomatoes are roasting, prepare the cauliflower rice. Place the cauliflower into a food processor and pulse until reduced to the size of rice grains.

Melt the coconut oil in a nonstick skillet over medium heat. Add the onion and cook for 5-6 minutes until translucent. Stir in the cauliflower, season with low sodium salt and pepper, and cover. Cook for 7-10 minutes until the cauliflower has softened, and then toss with parsley.

To make the lamb, preheat the oven to 325 degrees F. Pat the ostrich or venison dry and rub with olive oil. Generously season both sides with low sodium salt and pepper.

Heat one tablespoon of coconut oil in a cast iron skillet. When the pan is hot, add to the pan and sear for 2-3 minutes on all sides until golden brown.

Place the skillet in the oven and bake for 5-8 minutes until the ostrich or venison reaches desired doneness. Let rest for 10 minutes before serving.

While the meat is resting, add the red onion to the skillet with the pan drippings from the lamb. Sauté for 3-4 minutes, then add the white wine vinegar.

Turn the heat to high and cook until the vinegar has mostly evaporated. Add the stock and bring to a boil, cooking until the sauce reduces by half.

Stir in the mustard, and season to taste with low sodium salt and pepper. Pour over ostrich or venison to serve.

40. Tantalizing Turkey Pepper Stir-fry

Ingredients:
2 bell peppers, sliced
1 cup broccoli florets
2 cooked and shredded turkey breasts
1/4 teaspoon chili powder
low sodium salt and pepper to taste
1 tablespoon coconut oil for frying

Instructions:
Add 1 tablespoon coconut oil into a frying pan on a medium heat.

Place the sliced bell peppers into the frying pan.

After the bell peppers soften, add in the cooked turkey meat.

Add in the chili powder, low sodium salt and pepper.

Mix well and stir-fry for a few more minutes.

41. Cheeky Chicken Stir Fry

Ingredients:
1 pound boneless, skinless chicken breast
2 tablespoons coconut oil
1 medium onion, finely chopped (about 1 cup)
2 heads broccoli, sliced into 3-inch spears (about 4 cups)
2 medium carrots, sliced (about 1 cup)
2 heads baby bok choy, sliced crosswise into 1-inch strips (about 1½ cups)
4 ounces shiitake mushrooms, stemmed and thinly sliced (about 1 cup)
1 small zucchini, sliced (about 1 cup)
½ teaspoon low sodium salt
Garlic powder to taste
1½ cups water

Instructions:

Rinse the chicken and pat dry. Cut into 1-inch cubes and transfer to a plate.

Heat the coconut oil in a large skillet over medium heat

Saute the onion for 8 to 10 minutes, until soft and translucent

Add the broccoli, carrots, and chicken and saute for 10 minutes until almost tender

Add the bok choy, mushrooms, zucchini, and low sodium salt and saute for 5 minutes

Add 1 cup of the water, cover the skillet, and cook for about 10 minutes, until the vegetables are wilted

In a small bowl, dissolve the arrowroot powder in the remaining ½ cup of water, stirring until thoroughly combined

Season at the end with garlic powder, salt and if you like some chilli powder

42. Perfect Eastern Turkey Stir-Fry

Ingredients:
2 tbsp. of coconut oil
2 cloves of garlic (thinly sliced)
1 inch ginger (finely grated)
2-3 green (spring) onions (sliced into long slivers)
1 carrot (coarsely grated)
1 green pepper (sliced into thin, long pieces)
1 turkey breast (cut into bite-sized pieces)
1/4 cup water
2 tbsp. homemade veggie broth
A few drops of toasted sesame oil

Instructions:

Put a pot with a bit of low sodium salt to boil and make sure your rice noodles are handy. Later, when the water has boiled, pop the noodles in and give it a stir.

Heat 2 tbsp. coconut oil in a wok or large pan.

Add the sliced garlic and grated ginger to the wok and stir-fry for 30 seconds.

Add the green onion and stir-fry 1 more minute.

Add the carrot and stir-fry about a minute. You want it just barely cooked, not limp and soggy. Remove the vegetable mixture to a bowl and set aside.

Add another 2/3 tbsp. of coconut oil to the wok.

When the oil is very hot, add the green pepper and stir-fry for 1 minute.

Heat a ½ tbsp. of coconut oil, then add the pieces of turkey breast and stir-fry. I found that the turkey got some color from the previous ingredients that were in the wok. If this doesn't happen, add a tiny amount of soy sauce.

Stir-fry until just done and no more. To check, I like to cut open the biggest piece to make sure it isn't pink in the middle.

Add the sesame oil.

43. Creamy Curry Stir Fry

Ingredients:
2 cooked chicken breasts (small) or 3-4 thighs/legs
3 carrots, chopped
3 sticks celery, chopped
1-2 heads broccoli, chopped
1/2 medium onion, chopped
2 cloves garlic 1/2c coconut milk
1/2c almond or coconut milk
2 tbsp turmeric
2 tbsp curry powder
2 tbsp coconut oil

Instructions:
Put coconut oil in pan and add chopped onion. Cook until onion softens up, add garlic and cook for an additional few minutes.

Next up, add in the carrots, celery, and broccoli. Cook until they have softened a bit (but are not fully cooked).

Shred the cooked chicken up into small pieces for the stir fry and add the coconut milk, other milk, and curry spices.

Stir everything thoroughly, simmer for 5-10 minutes or until everything is cooked to your liking, and serve hot.

Add cauliflower rice (grated cauliflower boiled for 3 minutes)

44. Sexy Turkey Scramble

Ingredients:
1 pound ground turkey
2 medium yellow onions
2 bell peppers (any color)
2 medium squash or zucchini
1 large hand-full of fresh spinach (2-3 ounces)
Spices to taste: I used about 1 tablespoon each of: cumin, chili powder, garlic powder, low sodium salt, and fresh cilantro

Instructions:
Brown the turkey until well cooked in a large skillet or wok over medium high heat.

Remove and add thinly sliced onions, peppers, squash/zucchini to the pan and saute, stirring constantly, until starting to soften.

Return turkey to pan and add fresh spinach.

Spice to taste and continue to cook until spinach is wilted.

Remove and serve with any desired toppings.

45. Turkey Thai Basil

Ingredients:
2 lbs. leftover cooked turkey, cubed or shredded (chicken or shrimp would work too)
3 Tbsp fish sauce
3 Tbsp coconut aminos (or wheat free tamari)
1 Tbsp water
Stevia to taste
1 tsp low sodium salt
1/2 tsp ground white pepper
2 Tbsp coconut oil
4 baby bok choy, leaves pulled apart, hearts halved
1 red bell pepper, sliced
1 yellow bell pepper, sliced
1 large onion, sliced
3 cloves garlic, minced
1 1/2 C lightly pack Thai basil leaves

Instructions:

In a medium bowl, combine turkey with fish sauce, water, low sodium salt and pepper; stir until turkey is thoroughly coated and set aside

Melt coconut oil in large wok or frying pan over medium-high heat

Add bok choy, peppers, onion and garlic and saute until softened, about 8 minutes, stirring frequently

Add contents of set-aside bowl (with the meat) to pan and stir for about 3 minutes until turkey is fully incorporated and heated through

Remove from heat and add Thai basil, stirring until basil wilts

46. Chicken Fennel Stir-Fry

Ingredients:
3 chicken breasts or the meat from 1 whole roasted chicken
2 tablespoons coconut oil
1 onion
1 bulb of fennel
1 teaspoon each of low sodium salt, pepper, garlic powder and basil

Instructions:
Stovetop:

Cut the chicken into bite sized pieces. If chicken is raw, heat butter/coconut oil in large skillet or wok until melted.

Add chicken and cook on medium/high heat until chicken is cooked through. (If chicken is pre-cooked, cook the vegetables first then add chicken)

While cooking, cut the onion into bite sized pieces (1/2 inch) and thinly slice the fennel bulb into thin slivers.

Add all to skillet or wok, add spices and continue sautéing until all are cooked through and fragrant.

This will take approximately 10-12 minutes.

47. Moroccan Madness

Ingredients:
1 chicken breast, chopped into pieces
1/2 tbsp olive oil
1/2 onion, chopped
1 bell pepper, chopped
1 cup diced courgette
2 cloves garlic, minced
1 tsp ginger, minced
1 tsp cumin
1 tsp turmeric
1/2 tsp paprika
1/2 tbsp oregano
1/2 can diced tomatoes
1/2 cup low sodium chicken stock
low sodium salt and pepper

Instructions:
In a pan cook the chicken in the olive oil

Once it's finished cooking, remove from pan and set aside

Add to the pan the bell pepper, onion, courgette, garlic, ginger and all spices, sauté until bell pepper and onion become soft

Add back in the chicken along with the diced tomatoes and chicken stock, let simmer for 1o minutes

48. Thai Baked Fish with Squash Noodles

Ingredients:
1 medium spaghetti squash
Extra virgin olive oil, for drizzling
low sodium salt and pepper
1 tbsp coconut oil
1/2 large onion, finely chopped
1 head broccoli, de-stemmed and cut into florets
2 heads baby bok choy, sliced into 1-inch strips
4 scallions, sliced
1/4 tsp red pepper flakes
1/3 cup cashews, toasted and chopped

For the Sauce:
1 tsp lime juice
1/2-inch piece fresh ginger, peeled and minced
1 clove garlic, minced
1/2 tsp red wine vinegar
3 tbsp almond butter
3 tbsp coconut milk

For the Fish:
2 whole fish fillets…use cod or any good quality white fish

Instructions:

Preheat the oven to 400 degrees F. Place squash in the microwave for 3-4 minutes to soften. Using a sharp knife, cut the squash in half lengthwise. Scoop out the seeds and discard. Place the halves, with the cut side up, on a rimmed baking sheet. Drizzle with olive oil and sprinkle with low sodium salt and pepper. Roast in the oven for 45-50 minutes, until you can poke the squash easily with a fork. Let cool until you can handle it safely. Then scrape the insides with a fork to shred the squash into strands.

While the squash cooks, make the sauce. Combine the lime juice, ginger, garlic, and red wine vinegar in a blender or food processor until smooth. Add the almond butter and coconut milk and blend until completely combined. Adjust the levels of almond butter and coconut milk to reach desired level of creaminess.

Melt the coconut oil in a large pan over medium heat. Add the onion and cook for 5-6 minutes until translucent. Add the broccoli and sauté for 8-10 minutes, until just tender. Then stir in the bok choy and cook for 3-4 minutes until wilted. Lastly add the cooked spaghetti squash into the pan and stir to combine.

To assemble, top the spaghetti squash mixture with the scallions and cilantro. Sprinkle with roasted cashews and drizzle with Thai sauce.

Place the whole fish under the grill at 200 degrees for 25 minutes topped with a tablespoon of olive oil, fresh pressed garlic (one clove) and cayenne pepper to taste.

Finnish off the fish with a squirt of lemon juice to taste.

49. Divine Prawn Mexicana

Ingredients:
1 tbsp extra virgin olive oil
1 tsp chili powder
1 tsp low sodium salt
1 lb. medium shrimp, peeled and deveined
1 avocado, pitted and diced
Shredded lettuce, for serving
Fresh cilantro, for serving
1 lime, cut into wedges

For the tortillas:
6 egg whites
1/4 cup coconut flour
1/4 cup almond milk
1/2 tsp low sodium salt
1/2 tsp cumin
1/4 tsp chili powder

Instructions:

Combine all of the tortilla ingredients together in a small bowl and mix well. Allow the batter to sit for approximately 10 minutes to allow the flour to soak up some of the moisture, and then stir again. The consistency should be similar to crepe batter.

While the batter is resting, heat a skillet to medium-high. Mix together the olive oil, chili powder, and low sodium salt and toss with the shrimp to coat. Cook in the skillet for 1-2 minutes per side, until translucent. Set aside.

Coat the pan with coconut oil spray. Pour about 1/4 cup of batter onto the skillet, turning the pan with your wrist to help it spread out in a thin, even layer. Cook for 1-2 minutes, loosening the sides with a spatula. When the bottom has firmed up, carefully flip over and cook for another 2-3 minutes until lightly browned, then set aside on a plate. Repeat with remaining batter.

Top each tortilla with cooked shrimp, shredded lettuce, avocado, and cilantro. Serve with a lime wedge.

50. Superior Salmon with Lemon and Thyme OR Use any White fish

Ingredients:
32 oz piece of salmon or any fresh white fish
1 lemon, sliced thin
1 tbsp capers
low sodium salt and freshly ground pepper
1 tbsp fresh thyme
Olive oil

Instructions:
Line a rimmed baking sheet with parchment paper and place salmon, skin side down, on the prepared baking sheet.

Season salmon with low sodium salt and pepper. Arrange capers on the salmon, and top with sliced lemon and thyme.

Place baking sheet in a cold oven, then turn heat to 400 degrees F. Bake for 25 minutes. Serve immediately.

51. Spectacular Shrimp Scampi in Spaghetti Sauce

Ingredients:
For the Spaghetti:
1 spaghetti squash
Extra virgin olive oil, for drizzling
low sodium salt and pepper
1 tsp dried oregano
1 tsp dried basil

For the shrimp scampi:
8 oz. shrimp, peeled and deveined
3 tbsp butter
1 tbsp extra virgin olive oil
2 cloves garlic, minced
Pinch of red pepper flakes
low sodium salt and pepper, to taste
1 tbsp fresh parsley, chopped
Juice of 1 lemon
Zest of half a lemon

Instructions:
Preheat the oven to 400 degrees F. Place squash in the microwave for 3-4 minutes to soften. Using a sharp knife, cut the squash in half lengthwise. Scoop out the seeds and discard. Place the halves, with the cut side up, on a rimmed baking sheet.

Drizzle with olive oil and sprinkle with seasonings. Roast in the oven for 45-50 minutes, until you can poke the squash easily with a fork.

Let it cool until you can handle it safely. Then scrape the insides with a fork to shred the squash into strands.

After removing spaghetti squash from the oven, melt the butter and olive oil in a skillet over medium heat.

Add in the garlic and sauté for 2-3 minutes. Then add in the shrimp, low sodium salt, pepper, and a pinch of red pepper flakes.

Cook for 5 minutes, until the shrimp is cooked through. Remove from heat and add in desired amount of cooked spaghetti squash. Toss with lemon juice and zest. Top with parsley.

52. Scrumptious Cod in Delish Sauce

Ingredients:
1 lb. cod fillets
1/3 cup almond flour
1/2 tsp low sodium salt
2-3 tbsp extra virgin olive oil
2 tbsp walnut oil, divided
3/4 cup low sodium chicken stock
3 tbsp lemon juice
1/4 cup capers, drained
2 tbsp fresh parsley, chopped

Instructions:
Stir the almond flour and low sodium salt together in a shallow bowl. Rinse off the fish and pat dry with a paper towel. Dredge the fish in the almond flour mixture to coat.

Heat enough olive oil to coat the bottom of a large skillet over medium-high heat along with one tablespoon walnut oil. Working in batches, add the cod and cook for 2-3 minutes per side to brown. Remove to a plate and set aside.

Add the chicken stock, lemon juice, and capers to the same skillet and scrape any browned bits off the bottom. Simmer to reduce the sauce by almost half. Remove from heat and stir in the remaining tablespoon of walnut oil.

To serve, divide the cod onto plates, drizzle with the sauce, and sprinkle with parsley.

53. Delish Baked dill Salmon

Ingredients:
2 6-oz. salmon fillets
2 zucchini, halved lengthwise and thinly sliced
1/4 red onion, thinly sliced
1 tsp fresh dill, chopped
2 slices lemon
1 tbsp fresh lemon juice
Extra virgin olive oil, for drizzling
low sodium salt and freshly
ground pepper

Instructions:
Preheat the oven to 350 degrees F. Prepare a baking tray

Place half of the zucchini, red onion, dill, and one lemon slice. Drizzle with olive oil and sprinkle with low sodium salt and pepper. Place a salmon fillet on top and drizzle with the lemon juice. Season with low sodium salt and pepper. Repeat with the remaining ingredients.

Bake for 15-20 minutes until the salmon is opaque.

54. Prawn garlic Fried "Rice"

Ingredients:
1 tbsp coconut oil
1 cup white onion, finely chopped
2 cloves garlic, minced
8 oz. prawns peeled and deveined
1 medium carrot, chopped
1/2 cup peas
2 cups cooked cauliflower rice
2 eggs, beaten
Low sodium salt and pepper, to taste

Instructions:
Heat a wok or large pan over medium-high heat. Melt the coconut oil and add the onion and garlic to the pan.

Cook for 3-4 minutes until the onion starts to soften. Add the shrimp and cook for 1 minute.

Add the carrot, peas, and bell pepper to the pan. Cook for 3-4 minutes, and then stir in the cauliflower rice.

Clear a circle in the center of the pan and pour in the beaten eggs. Stir to scramble the eggs and then combine with the other ingredients.

Season with low sodium salt and pepper to taste.

55. Lemon and Thyme Super Salmon

Ingredients:
32 oz piece of salmon
1 lemon, sliced thin
2 tspns lemon juice
Low sodium salt and freshly ground pepper
1 tbsp fresh thyme
Olive oil, for drizzling

Instructions:
Heat a wok or large pan over medium-high heat. Melt the coconut oil and add the onion and garlic to the pan.

Cook for 3-4 minutes until the onion starts to soften. Add the shrimp and cook for 1 minute.

Add the carrot, peas, and bell pepper to the pan. Cook for 3-4 minutes, and then stir in the cauliflower rice.

Clear a circle in the center of the pan and pour in the beaten eggs. Stir to scramble the eggs and then combine with the other ingredients.

Season with low sodium salt and pepper to taste.

56. Delicious Salmon in Herb Crust

Ingredients:
2 salmon fillets (approx. 300g)
1 small onion, peeled and quartered
2 garlic cloves, peeled
1 sprig lemongrass, coarsely chopped
2 cm piece of ginger root, peeled
1 red chili pepper

Instructions:
Line a rimmed baking sheet with parchment paper and place salmon, skin side down, on the prepared baking sheet.

Generously season salmon with low sodium salt and pepper and top with sliced lemon and thyme.

Place baking sheet in a cold oven, then turn heat to 400 degrees F. Bake for 25 minutes.

Add lemon juice and serve immediately.

57. Salmon Mustard Delish

Ingredients:
4 tsp mustard seed
1/2 tsp garlic powder
1/4 tsp low sodium salt
1/4 tsp black pepper
1/4 tsp dried dill
1 1/2 lb salmon

Instructions:
Preheat oven to 200 degrees Celsius. (390 F)

Start by making the herb crust: combine the onion, garlic, lemongrass, ginger in the smallest bowl of a food processor

Process into a coarse paste.

Put the salmon fillets in an oven dish and spread the herb paste on top.

Bake for approx. 12-15 minutes until done, depending on the thickness of your fillets.

Serve with veggies of your choice and enjoy!

58. Sexy Spicy Salmon

Ingredients:
For the Salmon:
4 6 ounce Sockeye Salmon Filets
½ teaspoon of Cinnamon
½ teaspoon of Coriander
½ teaspoon of Cumin
¼ teaspoon of Ground Cloves
¼ teaspoon of Cardamom
low sodium salt to taste
1 Tablespoon of coconut butter

For the Lime Mustard dressing:
¼ cup of olive oil
1 Tablespoon of Lime Juice
2 teaspoons of mustard powder
Pinch of low sodium salt

Instructions:
Preheat the oven to 425°F. Grind all of the spices together with a mortar and pestle until mustard seeds are cracked, most are powder, and everything is well blended.

Spread the mixture over the salmon evenly, and place on a baking pan with a non-stick rack.

Bake for 15 to 20 minutes, until the flesh flakes easily with a fork. If you prefer salmon that is medium-rare, 15 minutes should do the trick.

Enjoy with your favorite sautéed greens, or mixed salad.

59. Mouthwatering Stuffed Salmon

Ingredients:
1 lb wild Alaskan or sockeye salmon, cut into 2 pieces
6 oz raw shrimp, peeled, deveined and chopped
1 large egg
2 tbsp raw onions, chopped
2 tbsp Italian flat leaf parsley, chopped
2 tbsp almond meal (or almond flour)
2 tbsp coconut butter
1 clove garlic, minced
low sodium salt and pepper to taste

Instructions:
For the Salmon:
Preheat oven to 400F
Pat dry the salmon filets with a paper towel.
Combine the cinnamon, coriander, cumin, cloves, and cardamom. Sprinkle evenly over the salmon filet side.
Heat an oven safe skillet (preferably cast iron) to medium high heat. Test the heat by placing a drop of water. It should immediately evaporate.
Add the coconut butter and let it melt.
Place the salmon filet side down and let sear for about 1-2 minutes. Flip and sear on the skin side for 1 minute.
Place the skillet inside the oven, with the skin side down.
Bake at 400F for 6-7 minutes.

For the Lime Mustard Mayo:

Combine dressing, lime juice, low sodium salt, and mustard.

Dip with salmon and enjoy!

60. Spectacular Salmon

Ingredients:
For the salmon:
2 salmon fillets (6oz each)
1 heaping tablespoon coconut flour
2 tablespoons fresh parsley
1 tablespoon olive oil
1 tablespoon mustard powder
low sodium salt and pepper, to taste

For the salad:
2 cups any green leaf salad
¼ red onion, sliced thin
juice of 1 lemon
1 tablespoon white wine vinegar
1 tablespoon olive oil
low sodium salt and pepper, to taste

Instructions:
Preheat oven to 375F.

Mix the chopped raw shrimp, egg, onions, parsley, almond meal, 1tbsp coconut butter, garlic, low sodium salt and pepper. Set aside.

Lightly season the salmon pieces with low sodium salt and pepper. Heat a cast iron pan on high and add the rest of the lard. Pan sear the salmon 1-2 minutes per side.

Move the salmon to an ovenproof dish and top each piece with 2 tbsp (or more!) of the shrimp topping. Lightly brush the top with a little bit of lard and bake in the oven for 15 minutes.

Afterwards, set your oven to broil and cook for about 3 more minutes until the top becomes crispy.

61. Creamy Coconut Salmon

Ingredients:
1 pound wild salmon fillets
¼ tsp low sodium salt
¼ tsp freshly ground black pepper
2 tsp coconut oil
3 cloves fresh garlic (minced)
1 large shallot (minced)
1 lemon (juice and zest)
½ cup unsweetened full-fat coconut milk

Instructions:
Preheat oven to 450 degrees.

Place salmon fillets on a parchment or foil lined baking sheet.

Top your salmon off with olive oil and mustard powder and rub into your salmon.

In a small bowl, mix together your coconut flour, parsley, and low sodium salt and pepper.

Use a spoon to sprinkle on your toppings on your salmon and then your hand to pat into your salmon.

Place in oven for 10-15 minutes or until salmon is cooked to your preference. I cooked mine more on the medium rare side at 12 minutes.

While the salmon is cooking, mix together your salad ingredients.

When salmon is done, place salmon on top of salad and consume.

62. Salmon Dill Bonanza

Ingredients:
1 1/2 pounds wild salmon (I used sockeye)
zest of one lemon (about a tablespoon)
2 tablespoons oil
1 tablespoon chopped, fresh dill
1 lemon
low sodium salt and pepper

Instructions:
Preheat oven to 375°F.

Place salmon in a shallow baking dish and season with low sodium salt and pepper.

Heat coconut oil in a medium saute pan or cast iron skillet over medium heat. Add garlic and shallots and saute until tender and fragrant, 3-5 minutes.

Add lemon zest, lemon juice, and coconut milk, stirring to combine.

Bring to a low boil, then remove from heat.

Pour mixture over salmon. Bake, uncovered, for 10-20 minutes or until salmon flakes easily with a fork.

63. Sexy Shrimp Cocktail

Ingredients:
1 pound uncooked shrimp, peeled, deveined, and thawed if frozen
1 tablespoon olive oil
Low sodium salt and fresh ground pepper to taste
1 cup coconut cream and two tablespoon tomato paste
One teaspoon fresh pressed garlic
lemon wedges

Instructions:
Preheat oven to 400 degrees F.

Oil the bottom of a 9 x 13 baking dish.

Rinse the salmon and pat dry with paper towels. Sprinkle with low sodium salt and pepper and place in the prepared dish.

Mix together the oil (room temperature), lemon zest and dill.

Place about half the mixture on top of the seasoned salmon. You can spread the lemon dill mixture or leave it in dollops like this.

Bake for about 10-15 minutes. The salmon will continue cooking even after you take it out of the oven.

Add the remaining oil/dill/lemon zest mixture on top, add a squeeze of lemon juice.

64. Gambas al Ajillo--Sizzling Garlic Shrimp

Ingredients:
1/2 cup olive oil
10 cloves garlic, peeled and thinly sliced
1 pound raw shrimp, peeled, deveined, and tails removed, defrosted if frozen
Low sodium salt and pepper to taste
1/4 teaspoon paprika
Pinch or two of red pepper flakes, optional

Instructions:
Preheat oven to 425 degrees.

Toss shrimp with oil, low sodium salt and pepper and spread in single layer on rimmed baking sheet.

Roast, turning once, until shrimp is pink and just cooked through (about 5-10 minutes, depending on size of shrimp).

Serve chilled with the blend of coconut cream, tomato paste and pressed garlic…add black pepper and lemon wedges.

65. Garlic Lemon Shrimp Bonanza

Ingredients:
1 lb shrimp, deveined
3-4 cloves of garlic, chopped
1/2 fresh lemon juice
3 tbsp olive oil
1/8 of low sodium salt
Fresh ground pepper (to taste)
1 tbsp fresh parsley, chopped for garnish

Instructions:
Preheat the broiler, if using. Heat the olive oil in a heavy skillet over medium-low heat.

Add the garlic and saute, stirring frequently, for about five minutes, until the garlic is softened but not browned.

Add the shrimp, raise the heat to medium high, and sprinkle with low sodium salt, pepper, paprika, and red pepper.

Cook for three minutes on each side or until the shrimp are completely opaque. Serve hot.

66. Courgette Pesto and Shrimp

Ingredients:
For the Pesto Sauce:
A ton of Basil
Minced Garlic
Pine Nuts
low sodium salt & Pepper

For the Zinguine:
1 Small Zucchini
low sodium salt & Pepper to taste

For the Shrimp:
Shrimp (peeled & de-veined)

Instructions:
Heat pan to medium-high heat.

Add ghee and garlic. Saute for about a minute.

Add shrimp. Saute for about a minute on each side.

Add low sodium salt, pepper and lemon juice. Saute for another minute or so.

Remove from heat and dish onto a plate or bowl.

67. Easy Shrimp Stir Fry

Ingredients:
1lb of wild shrimp
1 Lemon
3 Cloves of garlic, minced
2 Tablespoons of olive oil
1/2 teaspoon of garlic power
1 Dash of red pepper flakes
4 Tablespoons of olive oil

Instructions:
Throw all ingredients in a mini food processor. Pulse until it's a paste that you think looks and smells delicious.

Use a vegetable peeler and peel the courgette right into the pan, then saute.

Stir in pesto sauce and low sodium salt /pepper when the zucchini linguine starts turning transparent.

In another smaller skillet, cook shrimp over medium heat for approximately 3 minutes per side.

68. Delectable Shrimp Scampi

Ingredients:
4 tsp olive oil
1 1/4 pounds med raw shrimp, peeled and deveined (tails left on)
6-8 garlic cloves, minced
1/2 cup low sodium chicken broth
1/4 cup fresh lemon juice
1/4 cup + 1 T minced parsley
1/4 tsp low sodium salt
1/4 tsp freshly ground pepper
4 lemon wedges

Instructions:
Peal shrimp and butterfly them (making a cut in the back and extracting the vein).

Place shrimp in marinade: 2 Tablespoons olive oil, lemon, garlic powder. Marinade anywhere from 15 minutes to hours (the more time, the better)

Heat 2 Tablespoons of oil in pan on medium to high heat.

Add shrimp and cook each side for 2-3 minutes. Drizzle with 1 Tablespoon of olive oil.

Top with low sodium salt, pepper, and red pepper flakes.

69. Citrus Shrimp Delux

Ingredients:
3/4 pounds peeled and deveined medium-large shrimp
1/2 Tbls almond meal
2 Tbls orange juice, fresh squeezed
1/2 Tbls rice vinegar
1 Tbls diced chillies
1 Tbls olive oil
1/2 Tbls fresh ginger, minced
2 garlic cloves, minced

Instructions:
In a large nonstick skillet, heat the oil. Saute the shrimp until just pink, about 2-3 minutes. Add the garlic and cook stirring constantly, about 30 seconds. With a slotted spoon transfer the shrimp to a platter and keep them warm.

In the skillet, combine the broth, lemon juice, 1/4 cup of the parsley, the low sodium salt and pepper; and bring it to a boil. Boil uncovered, until the sauce is reduced by half.

Spoon the sauce over the shrimp. Serve garnished with the lemon wedges and sprinkled with the remaining tablespoon of parsley.

70. Sexy Garlic Shrimp

Ingredients:
4-5 T olive oil
4 garlic cloves, minced
1 t red pepper flakes
1 t smoked paprika
1 lb medium shrimp, peeled and deveined
2 T fresh lime juice
2 Teaspoons jerez sherry
low sodium salt and pepper to taste

Instructions:
Place shrimp in bowl and toss with almond powder.

Make sure shrimp is evenly coated.

In a small bowl whisk together orange juice, , honey, rice vinegar and chili

Heat olive oil in a large non-stick skillet over medium-high heat. Add ginger and garlic. Stir until garlic becomes fragrant. This will only take 10-15 seconds.

Add shrimp and cook for 3 minutes. Add in sauce and cook for additional 2 minutes. Remove shrimp with a slotted spoon.

Continue stirring sauce for another 2-4 minutes until it thickens. Drizzle over shrimp. Serve on top of baby spinach or fried cauliflower rice.

71. Shrimp Cakes Delux

Ingredients:
2 cups of small prawns
2 eggs
fresh chives
1/2 tsp spicy chili powder
1/2 tsp ground coriander
1/2 tsp garlic powder
shredded coconut
1/2 tbsp coconut flour

Instructions:

In a saute pan over medium heat, warm the olive oil.

Combine all ingredients and blend slightly to get a smoother consistency – but not too much

Make mixture into little cakes – size is your preference

Increase the heat to high, add the shrimp cakes, and saute and turn until the shrimp cake is cooked through – about 3 minutes.

Season with low sodium salt and black pepper.

72. Shrimp Spinach Spectacular

Ingredients:
2 tablespoons olive oil
½ yellow onion – diced
1 cup green beans
2 cloves garlic minced
½ teaspoon chili powder
½ lime – juiced
1 pound raw wild shrimp – thawed, cleaned, and tails removed
1 – 6 oz. bag of baby spinach
low sodium salt and pepper to taste

Instructions:
Chop the shrimp,

Next, mix in the spices, chives, 1 egg and the coconut flour.

Set up 2 bowls, 1 with shredded coconut and the other with the 2nd egg, whisked.

Form cakes of the shrimp mix - cover them with the whisked egg and then with shredded coconut.

Cook them in coconut oil on both sides until brown.

Serve with vegetables of your choice, or fried cauliflower rice.

73. Prawn Salad Boats

Ingredients:
1 lb shrimp, cooked
1 medium tomato, diced
1 cucumber, peeled and diced
3 tablespoons olive oil
One tablespoon coconut cream
Juice of one lemon
1/2 tsp dried dill
1/2 tsp celery seed
1/4 tsp low sodium salt
1/4 tsp pepper
Endive or big lettuce leaf, for serving

Instructions:

In a large sauté pan, heat olive oil over medium heat. Add onion, beans, and sauté until tender – approximately 10 minutes.

Add garlic, lime juice, and chili powder and continue to cook for an additional 5 minutes.

Add spinach and shrimp. Continue to cook for approximately 7-10 more minutes until spinach has wilted and shrimp is done. Place mixture on large lettuce leaves and serve.

74. Cheeky Curry Shrimp

Ingredients:
1 lb raw, peeled, tail on shrimp
2 tsp curry powder
1 tsp garlic powder
1 tsp ground coriander
1/2 tsp ground ginger
low sodium salt and black pepper to taste

Instructions:
In a medium bowl, mix the coconut cream, and lemon juice until combined.

Add the shrimp, tomato, cucumbers, capers, and spices.

Mix until everything is incorporated. Add additional low sodium salt and pepper to taste. Serve in endive leaves.

75. Courgette Shrimp Noodles

Ingredients:
1 pound fresh shrimp, peeled and deveined
4-5 medium courgettes julienned very small, about the size of spaghetti
1 onion, chopped
2 cloves garlic, chopped
1 can diced tomatoes, with liquid (14 oz.)
2 cups fresh spinach
1/2 tsp red chili flake
1 tsp fresh oregano
1 tbsp fresh lemon juice
1 tbsp olive oil

Instructions:
Rinse shrimp under cold water and pat dry with a paper towel.

Place shrimp in a large Ziploc bag.

In a small mixing bowl, curry powder, coriander, garlic powder, ground ginger, low sodium salt, and pepper.

Pour spice mixture over shrimp, seal bag, and toss to evenly coat.

Place shrimp in the fridge and allow to marinate for at least an hour.

Preheat grill to high heat and place all vegetables to grill and crisp for about 15 minutes with 1 tblspn olive oil.

Then grill shrimp about 6 minutes

76. Sexy Shrimp on Sticks

Ingredients:
1/2 lb shrimp, peeled and deveined
1/4 cup coconut milk
1 tsp fish sauce
6 gloves garlic, chopped
1/4 tsp each turmeric, cumin, low sodium salt

Instructions:
Heat olive oil in a large pan over medium heat. Add garlic and spices

Add shrimp and coconut last. Low sodium salt and pepper to taste and serve with a fresh squeeze of lemon.

Serve along side your choice of vegetable or fried cauliflower rice.

77. Delicious Fish Stir Fry

Ingredients:
200 grams any white fish fillet (cut into pieces)
1 Tablespoon Coconut or Apple ciderVinegar
1/2 Teaspoon Ginger and Garlic fresh pressed
1 small onion (quartered)
1/2 Cup Bell Peppers de-seeded and cubed (Red or Yellow).
1/2 Cup Mushrooms (any kind)
2 to 3 stalks of scallions (cut into 1.5 inch length)
low sodium salt to taste
1 Teaspoon Chili powder (Optional)
1 Teaspoon Fish Sauce – low salt
1/2 Tablespoon Extra Virgin Olive Oil

Instructions:
Put a pot with a bit of low sodium salt to boil and make sure your rice noodles are handy. Later, when the water has boiled, pop the noodles in and give it a stir.

Heat 2 tbsp. coconut oil in a wok or large pan.

Add the sliced garlic and grated ginger to the wok and stir-fry for 30 seconds.

Add the green onion and stir-fry 1 more minute.

Add the peppers and stir-fry about a minute. You want it just barely cooked, not limp and soggy. Remove the vegetable mixture to a bowl and set aside.

Add another 2/3 tbsp. of coconut oil to the wok.

When the oil is very hot, add the green pepper and stir-fry for 1 minute.

Heat a ½ tbsp. of coconut oil, then add the pieces of fish and stir-fry. Stir-fry until just done and no more. To check, I like to cut open the biggest piece to make sure it isn't raw in the middle.

Add the sesame oil.

78. Sexy Shrimp with Delish Veggie Stir Fry

Ingredients:
1 1/2 pounds of shrimp
1 tsp. of coconut oil
1/2 cup of thinly sliced onion
1/2 red bell pepper. thinly sliced
1 cup of full fat coconut milk
2 tbsp. fish sauce
1 tbsp curry powder
2 tbsp. of chopped cilantro

Instructions:
In a large bowl mix fish sauce, garlic and ginger.

Heat the olive oil in a wok (or a large nonstick skillet) over medium-high heat.

Once it starts to shimmer add onion and chillies. Stir-fry the onions until they start to brown around the edges, about 2 minutes.

Stir in the bok choy stems and stir-fry for 1 minute.

Add the beaten eggs and cook until it's nearly cooked through about 2 minutes, stirring often.

Stir in bok choy greens, basil and lime juice. And stir-fry for 30 seconds or so, until the greens are wilted. Serve immediately.

79. Skinny Delicious Slaw

Ingredients:
1/2 head of cabbage   (mix purple and white)
3 or 4 carrots
1 onion
3 tablespoons walnut oil
1 egg beaten
Stevia and low sdium salt to taste
1 Tbsp. fresh lemon juice
pepper to taste

Instructions:
Grate cabbage, carrots and onion and mix together.

Make dressing by mixing

beaten egg, walnut oil, lemon juice, and seasonings.

Chill and serve.

80.   Turkey Eastern Surprise

Ingredients:
For the salad:
2 cups grilled turkey, chopped
6 baby bok choy, grilled & chopped
2 green onions, chopped
1/4 cup cilantro, chopped
1 Tbl sesame seeds

For the dressing:
1 Tbl fresh ginger, chopped
2 Tbl coconut cream
1 Tbl fish sauce
1 Tbl sesame oil
2 Tbl fresh lime juice
1 tsp stevia powder or to taste

Instructions:
Combine all of the salad ingredients until well mixed.

Add all of the ingredients for the dressing into a blender or food processor, and blend until mostly smooth – there may be some small chunks of ginger left, that's ok.

Pour the dressing over the salad and toss lightly until coated.

Garnish with more sesame seeds if desired.

If possible let it sit for an hour in the fridge before serving so the flavors can really meld together.

81. Mediterranean Turkey Delish Salad

Ingredients:
1 roasted turkey (organic, soy-free and pastured is best)
1/2 cup of olive oil
1/4 cup fresh cilantro, chopped
1 head of romaine or butter lettuce
1 red onion, diced
1 lemon, juiced
low sodium salt and pepper as desired

Instructions:
Shred the turkey with your hands or chop up and put it in a big bowl.

Add the oil, red onion, cilantro, lemon, low sodium salt and pepper.

Mix well and serve on a lettuce boat.

82. Skinny Delicious Turkey Divine

Ingredients:
2/3 cup fresh lime juice
1/3 cup fish sauce
Stevia to taste
3/4 cup chicken stock low sodium
1 1/2 pounds ground turkey
1 cup thinly sliced green onions
3/4 cup thinly sliced shallots
3 tablespoons minced lemongrass
1 tablespoon thinly sliced serrano chile
1/2 cup chopped cilantro leaves
1/3 cup chopped mint leaves
low sodium salt
1 head of any lettuce

Instructions:
Whisk together lime juice, fish sauce, honey and chile-garlic sauce. Set aside.

Warm chicken stock in a medium heavy-bottomed pot over medium heat until simmering. Add ground turkey and simmer until cooked through. As the turkey is cooking, stir occasionally to break up the meat. This should take 6 to 8 minutes.

Add green onion, shallot, lemongrass and chiles, stirring to combine. Continue cooking until shallots turn translucent, stirring occasionally (about 4 minutes). Remove from the heat and drain off any liquid in the pot

Stir in lime juice-fish sauce mixture, cilantro and mint. Season to taste with low sodium salt (not much is needed if any).

Transfer mixture to a large bowl and serve beside a pile of lettuce leaves. Using a spoon, scoop on to the lettuce leaves and enjoy!

83. Chicken Basil Avo Salad

Ingredients:
2 boneless, skinless chicken breasts (organic, cooked and shredded)
1/2 cup fresh basil leaves, stems removed
1 cup sliced cherry tomatoes
2 small or 1 large ripe avocado, pits and skin removed
2 Tbsp. extra virgin olive oil
1/2 tsp. low sodium salt (or more to taste)
1/8 tsp. ground black pepper (or more to taste)

Instructions:
Place the cooked shredded chicken in a medium sized mixing bowl.

Place the basil, avocado, olive oil, low sodium salt and ground black pepper in a food processor and blend until smooth. You may need to scrape the sides a couple times to incorporate.

Pour the avocado and basil mixture into the mixing bowl with the shredded chicken and tomatoes and toss well to coat.

Taste and add additional low sodium salt and ground black pepper if desired. Keep in the fridge until ready to serve.

84. Skinny Chicken salad

Ingredients:
Salad:
1 small head (or 4 cups) savoy cabbage, finely shredded –
1 cup carrot, julienned
1/4 cup scallions, trimmed and julienned
1/4 cup radishes, julienned
1/4 cup fresh cilantro, chopped
1/4 cup fresh mint, chopped
2 cups cooked organic chicken

Vinaigrette:
2 tablespoons coconut or rice vinegar
2 tablespoons sesame oil (use unrefined or cold-pressed)
juice of 1/2 a lime
1 chipotle pepper – optional
1 clove garlic, crushed
1 teaspoon fresh ginger, grated

Instructions:
Salad – Combine cabbage, carrots, scallions and radishes. Top with chicken, cilantro and mint and set aside.

Vinaigrette –Combine the vinaigrette ingredients. Taste to see if it needs any adjustments. If it is too spicy, you can add more lime juice to counteract it.

Drizzle salad with vinaigrette & enjoy.

85. Turkey Taco Salad

Ingredients:
1/2 lbs (ish) leftover turkey, cooked and chopped
1 1/2 Tbsp taco seasoning (recipe follows)
1 tblsp. coconut or olive oil and 1 tblsp rice vinegar
1/4 c. water
Shredded lettuce

Optional Toppings - sliced olives, tomatoes, red onion, avocado, bell peppers, crushed sweet potato chips

Taco Seasoning:
Mix together, 4 Tbsp. chili powder, 1 tsp each garlic powder, onion powder, and oregano, 2 tsp each paprika and cumin, 4 tsp low sodium salt, and 1/8-1/4 tsp red pepper flakes.

Instructions:

In a skillet, heat 1 teaspoon oil and add in chicken - I like to fry it for a minute to give some extra flavor. Add in water and taco seasoning, let simmer until liquid is gone.

Meanwhile, shred, chop, and dice all your toppings.

Assemble, lettuce, optional toppings, chicken, leftover oil and vinegar dressing, and crushed chips.

86. Cheeky Turkey Salad

Ingredients:
For the Turkey:
1 lb boneless turkey breasts
1 tbsp olive oil
low sodium salt and pepper, to taste

For the Salsa:
1 large tomato, quartered
1/2 red onion, cut into large chunks
1 garlic clove, peeled
1 small bunch of cilantro leaves
Juice of 1 lime
low sodium salt and pepper, to taste

Instructions:
Preheat oven to 375 F.

Bake turkey breasts dipped in olive oil on a baking sheet for 35 to 40 minutes, until no longer pink in the center.

While baking, add all salsa ingredients to a food processor and pulse using the chopping blade until finely chopped. Transfer the salsa to a large bowl and clean out the food processor. You will be using it to shred the turkey.

(If you don't have a food processor, just dice the tomato, onion, pepper, cilantro and garlic and add to a bowl with the lime juice, low sodium salt and pepper).

Remove turkey from the oven and allow to cool. Once cool enough to handle, cut each breast into three or four smaller pieces and add to the food processor. Pulse using the chopping blade until shredded.

Add turkey to bowl with salsa and mix well with a fork.

Refrigerate for at least two hours until turkey salad is chilled.

87. Macadamia Chicken Salad

Ingredients:
1lb organic chicken breast
1tsp macadamia nut oil, or oil of choice
few pinches of low sodium salt and pepper
1/2 cup macadamia nuts, chopped
1/2 cup diced celery
2 tbsp julienned basil
1 tablespoon olive oil and 2 teaspoons rice vinegar
1 tbsp lemon juice

Instructions:
Preheat oven to 350. Place chicken breasts on sheet tray, drizzle will oil and a pinch of low sodium salt and pepper. Bake for about 35 minutes until cooked through. Remove from oven and let cool.

In a large bowl shred chicken. Add nuts, celery, basil, dressing, and a pinch of low sodium salt and pepper. Gently stir until combined. Eat!

88. Rosy Chicken Supreme Salad

Ingredients:
For the chicken:
450g chicken mince, free range of course
1 long red chili, finely chopped with the seeds
2 garlic cloves, finely chopped
Little nob of fresh ginger, peeled and finely chopped
1 stem lemon grass, pale section only, finely chopped
1/2 bunch of coriander stems washed and finely chopped (I don't waste anything, save the leaves for the salad)
2 1/2 tbsp fish sauce
1/2 lime rind grated
1/2 lime, juiced
A pinch of low sodium salt
Coconut oil for frying (about 3 tablespoons)

For the salad:
1/4 red cabbage, thinly sliced
1 large carrot, peeled and grated
1/2 Spanish onion, thinly sliced
2 tbsp green spring onion, chopped
1/2 bunch of fresh coriander leaves (saved from the stems used in the chicken)
A handful of fresh mint or Thai basil if available
1/2 cup crashed roasted cashews or some sesame seeds

For the dressing:
2 tbsp olive oil
3 tbsp lime juice
1 tbsp fish sauce
1 small red chili, finely chopped

Instructions:
Once you've prepared all your ingredients for the chicken, heat 1 tbsp of coconut oil in a large frying pan or a wok to high.

Throw in lemongrass, chili, garlic, coriander stems and ginger and stir fry for about a minute until fragrant.

Add chicken mince and lime zest. Stir and break apart the mince with a wooden mixing spoon until separated into small chunks (this might take a while as chicken mince is quite sticky).

The meat will now be changing to white colour.

Add fish sauce and lime juice. Stir through and cook for a further few minutes. Total cooking time for the chicken should be about 10 minutes.

Prepare the salad base by mixing together sliced red cabbage, onion grated carrot, and fresh herbs.

Mix all dressing ingredients and toss through the salad.

Serve cooked chicken mince on top of the dressed salad and topped with roasted cashews, dried shallots, coconut flakes and extra fresh herbs.

89. Turkey Sprouts Salad

Ingredients:
1/2 pound of brussels sprouts (2-ish cups once sliced)
1/2 cup chopped almonds
2 turkey breasts, chopped
1/2 white onion, finely diced

Vinaigrette:
2 TBSP Apple Cider Vinegar
1 TBSP quality mustard powder
1 TBSP avocado oil
Stevia to taste
1/2 tsp low sodium salt
few grinds of black pepper

Instructions:
Cut the brussels sprouts in half and thinly slice. Chop the half cup of almonds. Finely dice the white onion. Scallions would work too if you prefer a more mild onion flavor… though the white did not overpower.

Remove the breasts and chop into bite-sized pieces. Combine all of these ingredients into a large bowl and gently toss the Brussels sprouts salad.

Whipping up the vinaigrette takes seconds. Add all ingredients to a small bowl and whisk until smooth. Pour over the Brussels sprouts salad and toss to bring together.

90. Delicious Chicken Salad

Ingredients:
Cooked and chopped chicken breast
Chopped almonds
Mashed avocado
Lots of low sodium salt and pepper
Any lettuce leaves of choice

Instructions:
Mix the first six ingredients together in a bowl, season with low sodium salt and pepper, and then spoon onto lettuce leaves. Roll up and enjoy!

91. Avocado Tuna Salad

Ingredients:
2 tins high quality albacore tuna
1 avocado
1/4 of an onion, chopped
juice of 1/2 a lime
2 Tbsp cilantro (or sub basil if you prefer)
some low sodium salt and pepper, to taste

Instructions:
Shred the tuna.

Add all of the other ingredients and mix.

92. Classic Tuna Salad

Ingredients:
2 large grilled tuna steaks
2 tablespoons olive oil
.5 cup onion, chopped (I like red, scallions are also good)
2-3 stalks celery, chopped (or .5 cup)
.5 – .75 cup pecans, chopped (optional)
.5 – 1 tsp low sodium salt
.5 tsp Lemon Garlic pepper
.5 – 1 Tbsp lemon juice

Instructions:
Grill the tuna steaks medium rare with garlic powder and black pepper to taste

Then do a bunch of chopping. Onions, celery, and pecans.

Combine all of these ingredients in the bowl with your cubed tuna and then start adding the dressing of oil and lemon juice seasoned.

You want enough to cover all the ingredients and make them moist, but not overly runny or dry.

It tastes great served right away, but even better after it sits in the fridge for a day.

93. Artichoke Tuna Delight

Ingredients:
1.5 cups diced grilled tuna
¼ cup finely diced red onion
1 small carrot julienned and cut into small pieces (or ½ a diced red bell pepper)
4-5 artichoke hearts (I used canned in water) diced
2 tablespoons capers
low sodium salt and pepper to taste.
6 Radicchio leaves

Instructions:
Place all ingredients, except the radicchio leaves in a large bowl and combine.

Place a scoop if salad into each Radicchio cup and serve.

Store salad in an air tight container in the fridge.

94. Tasty Tuna Stuffed Tomato

Ingredients:
2 large tomatoes
Lettuce leaves (optional)
2 (5 or 6 oz.) cans wild albacore tuna
6 Tbsp. olive oil and 1 tablespoon rice vinegar
1 stalk celery, chopped
1/2 small onion, chopped
1/4 tsp. low sodium salt
1/4 tsp. ground black pepper

Instructions:
Wash and dry the tomatoes and remove any stem. You can either slice off the top part of the tomatoes and hollow them out, or cut each tomato into wedges, making sure to only cut down to about 1/2 inch before you get to the bottom of the tomato.

Arrange the tomatoes on a plate on top of lettuce leaves (optional).

Combine the remaining ingredients in a mixing bowl and add additional low sodium salt and/or pepper if desired. Spoon into the tomatoes and serve.

95. Advanced Avocado Tuna Salad

Ingredients:
1 avocado
1 lemon, juiced, to taste
1 tablespoon chopped onion, to taste
1 cup chopped tomatoes
5 ounces cooked or canned wild tuna
low sodium salt and pepper to taste

Instructions:
Cut the avocado in half and scoop the middle of both avocado halves into a bowl, leaving a shell of avocado flesh about 1/4-inch thick on each half.

Add lemon juice and onion to the avocado in the bowl and mash together.

Add tuna, low sodium salt and pepper, and stir to combine. Taste and adjust if needed.

Fill avocado shells with tuna salad and serve.

96. Sexy Italian Tuna Salad

Ingredients:
10 sun-dried tomatoes
2 (5 oz) can of tuna
1-2 ribs of celery, diced finely
2 Tablespoons of extra virgin olive oil
1 cloves garlic, minced
3 Tablespoons finely chopped parsley
1/2 Tablespoon lemon juice
low sodium salt and pepper to taste

Instructions:

Prepare the sun-dried tomatoes by softening them in warm water for 30 minutes until soft. Then, pat the tomatoes dry and chop finely.

Flake the tuna.

Mix the tuna together with the chopped tomatoes, celery, extra virgin olive oil, garlic, parsley, and lemon juice. Add low sodium salt and pepper to taste.

If not serving immediately, mix with extra olive oil just before serving.

Optional: Make cucumber boats with them.

97. Divine Chicken or Turkey and Baby Bok Choy Salad

Ingredients:
For the salad:
2 cups grilled chicken or turkey, chopped
6 baby bok choy, grilled & chopped
2 green onions, chopped
1/4 cup cilantro, chopped
1 Tbl sesame seeds

For the dressing:
1 Tbl fresh ginger, chopped
2 Tbl coconut cream
1 Tbl sesame oil
2 Tbl fresh lime juice
1 tsp stevia powder

Instructions:
Combine all of the salad ingredients until well mixed.

Add all of the ingredients for the dressing into a blender or food processor, and blend until mostly smooth

Pour the dressing over the salad and toss lightly until coated.

Garnish with more sesame seeds if desired.

98. Mediterranean Medley Salad

Ingredients:
1 roasted chicken (organic, soy-free and pastured is best).. or turkey or ostrich steak

Dressing:
1/2 cup of olive oil, ¼ cup applecider vinegar and garlick powder and chilli powder to taste
1/4 cup fresh cilantro, chopped
1 head of romaine or butter lettuce
1 red onion, diced
1 lemon, juiced
low sodium salt and pepper as desired

Instructions:
Shred the chicken/turkey etc or chop up and put it in a big bowl.

Add the dressing…also red onion, cilantro, lemon, low sodium salt and pepper.

Mix well and serve on a lettuce boat.

99. Spicy Eastern Salad

Ingredients:
2/3 cup fresh lime juice
1/3 cup fish sauce(optional)
Stevia to taste
3/4 cup low sodium chicken stock (preferably homemade)
1 1/2 pounds ground chicken or turkey
1 cup thinly sliced green onions
3/4 cup thinly sliced shallots
3 tablespoons minced lemongrass
1 tablespoon thinly sliced serrano or other chile - optional
1/2 cup chopped cilantro leaves
1/3 cup chopped mint leaves
low sodium salt
1 head of butter lettuce or other green leaves

Instructions:

Whisk together lime juice, fish sauce (optional – try low sodium version)..stevia and Set aside.

Warm chicken stock in a medium heavy-bottomed pot over medium heat until simmering.

Add ground chicken and simmer until cooked through. As the chicken is cooking, stir occasionally to break up the meat. This should take 6 to 8 minutes.

Add green onion, shallot, lemongrass and chiles, stirring to combine. Continue cooking until shallots turn translucent, stirring occasionally (about 4 minutes).

Remove from the heat and drain off any liquid in the pot. I do this by clamping the lid on, then cracking it just a hair. I turn the entire pot over the sink and let the liquid drain out.

Stir in lime juice-fish sauce mixture, cilantro and mint. Season to taste with low sodium salt (not much is needed if any).

Transfer mixture to a large bowl and serve beside a pile of lettuce leaves. Using a slotted spoon, scoop on to the lettuce leaves and enjoy!

100. Basil Avocado Bonanza Salad

Ingredients:
2 boneless, skinless chicken or turkey breasts (cooked and shredded)
1/2 cup fresh basil leaves, stems removed
2 small or 1 large ripe avocado, pits and skin removed
2 Tbsp. extra virgin olive oil
1/2 tsp. low sodium salt (or more to taste)
1/8 tsp. ground black pepper (or more to taste)

Instructions:
Place the cooked shredded chicken in a medium sized mixing bowl.

Place the basil, avocado, olive oil, low sodium salt and ground black pepper in a food processor and blend until smooth.

Pour the avocado and basil mixture into the mixing bowl with the shredded chicken and toss well to coat.

Taste and add additional low sodium salt and ground black pepper if desired. Keep in the fridge until ready to serve.

101. Chinese Divine Salad

Ingredients:

Salad :
1 small head (or 4 cups) savoy cabbage, finely shredded –
1 cup carrot, julienned (about 1 large carrot)
1/4 cup scallions, trimmed and julienned (about 3 scallions)
1/4 cup radishes, julienned
1/4 cup fresh cilantro, chopped
1/4 cup fresh mint, chopped
2 cups cooked chicken or turkey

Vinaigrette:
2 tablespoons coconut or rice vinegar
Low sodium salt to taste
2 tablespoons sesame oil
1 chipotle pepper
1/2 teaspoon chilli flakes
1 clove garlic, crushed
1 teaspoon fresh ginger, grated
Stevia to taste

Instructions:

Salad – Combine cabbage, carrots, scallions and radishes. Top with chicken, cilantro and mint and set aside.

Vinaigrette –Combine the vinaigrette ingredients. Taste to see if it needs any adjustments. If it is too spicy, you can add more lime juice to counteract it.

Drizzle salad with vinaigrette & enjoy

102. Divinely Delish Salad Surprise

Ingredients:
1/2 lbs (ish) leftover chicken, turkey or boiled egg cooked and chopped
1 tsp. coconut or olive oil
1/4 c. water
Shredded lettuce
Optional Toppings - sliced olives, tomatoes, red onion, avocado, bell peppers
Non-optional Toppings - crushed sweet potato chips

Divine Dressing:
Mix together, 4 Tbsp. chili powder, 1 tsp each garlic powder, onion powder, and oregano, 2 tsp each paprika and cumin, 4 tsp low sodium salt, and 1/8-1/4 tsp red pepper flakes. Add 1 cup olive oil and half cup rice vinegar

Instructions:
Then, in a skillet, heat the oil and add in chicken etc –. Add in water let simmer until liquid is gone.

Meanwhile, shred, chop, and dice all your toppings.

Assemble, lettuce, optional toppings, chicken, dressing, and crushed chips.

Add Divine Dressing.

103. Avocado Salad with Cilantro and Lime

Ingredients:
Turkey Breast chopped
Two avocados, diced
2/3 green cabbage, chopped
5 green onions (scallions), white and pale green parts, minced
Juice of 2 limes
Two handfuls of fresh cilantro, chopped
low sodium salt to taste
One large English Cucumber

Instructions:
Mix all ingredients except cucumber -slice it thinly and use it as a base for the salad. For "party style", slice 1-2 inch sections, scoop out the center with a grapefruit spoon, and fill the cucumber "cups" with the salad.

Divine Dressing:
Mix together, 4 Tbsp. chili powder, 1 tsp each garlic powder, onion powder, and oregano, 2 tsp each paprika and cumin, 4 tsp low sodium salt, and 1/8-1/4 tsp red pepper flakes. Add 1 cup olive oil and half cup rice vinegar.

104. Mexican Medley Salad

Ingredients:

For the Chicken or turkey:
1 lb boneless chicken/turkey breasts
1 tbsp olive oil
low sodium salt and pepper, to taste

For the Salsa:
1 large tomato, quartered
1/2 red onion, cut into large chunks
1 jalapeno pepper, stem and seeds removed and halved
1 garlic clove, peeled
1 small bunch of cilantro leaves
Juice of 1 lime
low sodium salt and pepper, to taste

Instructions:
Preheat oven to 375 F.

Brush chicken breasts on both sides with olive oil and sprinkle with low sodium salt and pepper. Bake on a baking sheet for 35 to 40 minutes, until no longer pink in the center.

While chicken is baking, add all salsa ingredients to a food processor and pulse using the chopping blade until finely chopped.

Transfer the salsa to a large bowl and clean out the food processor. You will be using it to shred the chicken.

Remove chicken from the oven and allow to cool. Once cool enough to handle, cut each breast into three or four smaller pieces and add to the food processor. Pulse using the chopping blade until shredded.

Add chicken to bowl with salsa and mix well with a fork.

Refrigerate for at least two hours until chicken salad is chilled.

105. Macadamia Nut Chicken/Turkey Salad

Ingredients:
1lb chicken/turkey breast
1tsp macadamia nut oil, or oil of choice
few pinches of low sodium salt and pepper
1/2 cup macadamia nuts, chopped
1/2 cup diced celery
3 tbsp divine dressing
2 tbsp julienned basil
1 tbsp lemon juice

Instructions:
Preheat oven to 350. Place chicken breasts on sheet tray, drizzle will oil and a pinch of low sodium salt and pepper.

Bake for about 35 minutes until cooked through. Remove from oven and let cool.

In a large bowl shred chicken. Add nuts, celery, basil, mayo, lemon juice, and a pinch of low sodium salt and pepper. Gently stir until combined. Eat!

Divine Dressing:
Mix together, 4 Tbsp. chili powder, 1 tsp each garlic powder, onion powder, and oregano, 2 tsp each paprika and cumin, 4 tsp low sodium salt, and 1/8-1/4 tsp red pepper flakes. Add 1 cup olive oil and half cup rice vinegar.

106. Red Cabbage Bonanza Salad

Ingredients:

For the chicken or turkey:
450g chicken/turkey mince, free range of course
1 long red chili, finely chopped with the seeds
2 garlic cloves, finely chopped
Little nob of fresh ginger, peeled and finely chopped
1 stem lemon grass, pale section only, finely chopped
1/2 bunch of coriander stems washed and finely chopped (I don't waste anything, save the leaves for the salad)
1 tbs low sodium salt
1 tbsp coconut aminos
1/2 lime rind grated
1/2 lime, juiced
A pinch of low sodium salt
Coconut oil for frying (about 3 tablespoons)

For the salad:
1/4 red cabbage, thinly sliced
1 large carrot, peeled and grated
1/2 Spanish onion, thinly sliced
2 tbsp green spring onion, chopped
1/2 bunch of fresh coriander leaves (saved from the stems used in the chicken)
A handful of fresh mint or Thai basil if available
1/2 cup crashed roasted cashews or some seasame seeds
1/2 cup dried fried shallots (optional for garnish)
2 tbsp toasted coconut flakes (optional for garnish)

For the dressing:
2 tbsp olive oil
3 tbsp lime juice
1 small red chili, finely chopped (you can leave it out if you like it mild)

Instructions:

Once you've prepared all your ingredients for the chicken, heat 1 tbsp of coconut oil in a large frying pan or a wok to high. Throw in lemongrass, chili, garlic, coriander stems and ginger and stir fry for about a minute until fragrant.

Add chicken mince and lime zest. Stir and break apart the mince with a wooden mixing spoon until separated into small

The meat will now be changing to white colour. Add lime juice. Stir through and cook for a further few minutes. Total cooking time for the chicken should be about 10 minutes.

Prepare the salad base by mixing together sliced red cabbage, onion grated carrot, and fresh herbs.

Mix all dressing ingredients and toss through the salad.

Serve cooked chicken mince on top of the dressed salad and topped with roasted cashews, dried shallots, coconut flakes and extra fresh herbs.

107. Spectacular Sprouts Salad

Ingredients:
1/2 pound of mixed sprouts (2-ish cups once sliced)
1/2 Granny Smith apple
1/2 cup chopped almonds
2 chicken breasts, chopped
1/2 white onion, finely diced

Vinaigrette:
2 TBSP Apple Cider Vinegar
1 TBSP quality brown mustard
1 TBSP avocado oil
Stevia to taste
1/2 tsp low sodium salt
few grinds of black pepper

Instructions:
Cut Granny Smith apple, slicing into matchsticks.

Chop the half cup of almonds. Finely dice the white onion. Scallions would work too if you prefer a more mild onion flavor… though the white did not overpower.

Remove the breasts and chop into bite-sized pieces. Combine all of these ingredients into a large bowl and gently toss the sprouts into the salad.

Whipping up the vinaigrette takes seconds. Add all ingredients to a small bowl and whisk until smooth. Pour over the sprouts salad and toss to bring together.

108. Avocado Egg Salad

Ingredients:
Cooked and chopped organic eggs x 3
Chopped almonds
Mashed avocado
low sodium salt and pepper
Any lettuce leaves

Instructions:
Mix the ingredients together in a bowl, season with low sodium salt and pepper, and then spoon onto lettuce leaves. Roll up and enjoy!

109. Avocado Divine Salad

Ingredients:
1 kilo boneless, skinless chicken or turkey breasts (2 or 3)
1 avocado
1/4 of an onion, chopped
juice of one lime and one lemon
2 Tbsp cilantro (or sub basil if you prefer)
some low sodium salt and pepper, to taste
One bag mixed lettuce leaves
One tablespoon olive oil

Instructions:
Cook chicken breast until done, let cool, and then shred. Add all of the other ingredients and mix.

110. Classic Waldorf Salad

Ingredients:
half whole cooked chicken or turkey (~2lbs)
half cup apple, peeled and chopped (optional)
half cup onion, chopped (I like red, scallions are also good)
2-3 stalks celery, chopped (or .5 cup)
half cup pecans, chopped (optional)
half tsp low sodium salt
half tsp Lemon Garlic
pepper
1 Tbsp lemon juice

Divine Dressing:
Mix together, 4 Tbsp. chili powder, 1 tsp each garlic powder, onion powder, and oregano, 2 tsp each paprika and cumin, 4 tsp low sodium salt, and 1/8-1/4 tsp red pepper flakes. Add 1 cup olive oil and half cup rice vinegar

Instructions:
First cook up a whole chicken. You can buy a rotisserie chicken, or do what I do, throw a chicken in the crockpot, sprinkle it with cumin, low sodium salt & pepper and let it cook for about 4-6 hours on low.

After the chicken is cooked and cooled, de-bone and shred the meat (white and dark) and put it in a large mixing bowl. I usually use about half of my 3-4lb chicken.

Then do a bunch of chopping. Peel your apple, then chop your apple, onions, celery, and pecans.

Combine all of these ingredients in the bowl with your chicken and then start adding the dressing. You want enough to cover all the ingredients and make them moist, but not overly runny or dry.

Add the low sodium salt and pepper, and lemon juice Stir well to combine. Add dressing.

111. Artichoke Heart & Turkey Salad Radicchio Cups

Ingredients:
1.5 cups diced cooked turkey
¼ cup finely diced red onion
1 small carrot julienned and cut into small pieces (or ½ a diced red bell pepper)
4-5 artichoke hearts (I used canned in water) diced low sodium salt and pepper to taste.
6 Radicchio leaves

Instructions:
Place all ingredients, except the radicchio leaves in a large bowl and combine.

Place a scoop if salad into each Radicchio cup and serve.

Store salad in an air tight container in the fridge.

Divine Dressing:
Mix together, 4 Tbsp. chili powder, 1 tsp each garlic powder, onion powder, and oregano, 2 tsp each paprika and cumin, 4 tsp low sodium salt, and 1/8-1/4 tsp red pepper flakes. Add 1 cup olive oil and half cup rice vinegar.

112. Tempting Tuna Stuffed Tomato

Ingredients:
2 large tomatoes
Lettuce leaves (optional)
2 (5 or 6 oz.) cans wild albacore tuna
1 stalk celery, chopped
1/2 small onion, chopped
1/4 tsp. low sodium salt
1/4 tsp. ground black pepper

Instructions:
Wash and dry the tomatoes and remove any stem.

Arrange the tomatoes on a plate on top of lettuce leaves (optional).

Combine the remaining ingredients in a mixing bowl and add additional low sodium salt and/or pepper if desired.

Spoon into the tomatoes and serve.

113. Incredibly Delish Avocado Tuna Salad

Ingredients:
1 avocado
1 lemon, juiced, to taste
1 tablespoon chopped onion, to taste
5 ounces cooked or canned wild tuna
low sodium salt and pepper to taste

Instructions:
Cut the avocado in half and scoop the middle of both avocado halves into a bowl, leaving a shell of avocado flesh about 1/4-inch thick on each half.

Add lemon juice and onion to the avocado in the bowl and mash together. Add tuna, low sodium salt and pepper, and stir to combine. Taste and adjust if needed.

Fill avocado shells with tuna salad and serve.

114. Italian Tuna Bonanza Salad

Ingredients:
10 sun-dried tomatoes
2 (5 oz) can of tuna
1-2 ribs of celery, diced finely
2 Tablespoons of extra virgin olive oil
1 cloves garlic, minced
3 Tablespoons finely chopped parsley
1/2 Tablespoon lemon juice
low sodium salt and pepper to taste

Instructions:
Prepare the sun-dried tomatoes by softening them in warm water for 30 minutes until soft. Then, pat the tomatoes dry and chop finely.

Flake the tuna. and mix the tuna together with the chopped tomatoes, celery, extra virgin olive oil, garlic, parsley, and lemon juice. Add low sodium salt and pepper to taste.

If not serving immediately, mix with extra olive oil just before serving.

Optional: Make cucumber boats with them.

115. Asian Aspiration Salad

Ingredients:
1 red bell pepper, sliced
1 large carrot, cut into matchsticks
1 cucumber, halved lengthwise and sliced

Optional:
fresh ginger juice and rice vinegar
2 boiled eggs

Instructions:
Mix ingredients and Serve.

116. Tasty Carrot Salad

Ingredients:
5 carrots, medium
1 tbs. whole black mustard seeds
1/4 tsp. low sodium salt
2 tsp. lemon juice
2 tbs. olive oil
Add 1 Grated egg on top

Instructions:
Trim and peel and grate carrots. In a bowl, toss with low sodium salt and set aside.

In a small heavy pan over medium heat, heat oil.

When very hot, add mustard seeds. As soon as the seeds begin to pop, in a few seconds, pour oil and seeds over carrots.

Add lemon juice and toss. Serve at room temperature or cold.

Add Grated egg.

117. Creamy Carrot Salad

Ingredients:
1 pound carrots - shredded
20 ounces crushed pineapple -- drained
8 ounces Coconut milk
3/4 cup flaked coconut
Stevia to taste
Shredded turkey one breast

Instructions:
Combine all ingredients, tossing well. Cover and chill.

118. Vegetarian Curry with Squash

Ingredients:
1 tbsp coconut oil
2 cups mixed raw nuts.
1 medium yellow onion, diced
1 tsp low sodium salt
1 green bell pepper, thinly sliced
4 cloves garlic, minced
1-inch piece fresh ginger, peeled and minced
1 14-oz. can coconut milk
1 large acorn squash, peeled, seeded, and cut into 1-inch cubes
2 tsp lime juice
One teaspoon curry powder (mild or hot)
1/4 cup cilantro, chopped
Cauliflower rice, for serving

Instructions:

Melt the coconut oil in a large pan over medium heat. Add the onion and cook for 5-6 minutes, stirring occasionally. Add the bell pepper, garlic, ginger, and low sodium salt and stir to combine. Cook for an additional minute.

Add the curry powder to the pan and cook for about a minute, stirring to coat the other ingredients. Add in the coconut milk and bring to a simmer. Stir in the squash.

Simmer, stirring occasionally, for 15-20 minutes until the squash is fork-tender. Remove the pan from the heat and stir in the lime juice. Taste and adjust low sodium salt and lime juice as necessary. Sprinkle with cilantro to serve.

Roast the nuts under the grill until crisp and sprinkle over the top of the curry.

Serve with Cauliflower rice!

119. Saucy Gratin with Creamy Cauliflower Bonanza

Ingredients:
1 medium butternut squash, peeled, seeded, and diced
1 large sweet potato, peeled and thinly sliced
6 cups fresh spinach
1 tbsp extra virgin olive oil
2 large shallots, diced
4 cloves garlic, chopped
low sodium salt and pepper, to taste
Pinch of nutmeg

For the sauce:
1/2 head of cauliflower, cut into florets
1 cup almond milk
1/2 cup low sodium chicken stock
1/2 tsp low sodium salt
1/2 tsp freshly ground pepper
1/4 tsp nutmeg

Instructions:

Preheat the oven to 375 degrees F. To make the cream sauce, place a couple inches of water in a large pot. Once the water is boiling, place steamer insert and then cauliflower florets into the pot and cover. Steam for 12-14 minutes, until completely tender.

Drain and return cauliflower to the pot. Add the almond milk, stock, nutmeg, low sodium salt, and pepper to the pot. Use an immersion blender or food processor to combine the ingredients until smooth. Set aside.

Meanwhile, bring a separate pot of water to a boil. Add the butternut squash and cook for 4 minutes. Drain and set aside.

Heat the oil in a small pan over medium heat. Add the shallots and garlic and cook for 4-5 minutes until soft. Stir in the spinach to wilt. Season with low sodium salt and pepper.

To assemble, grease a large baking dish with coconut oil spray. Spoon a thin layer of the cream sauce over the bottom of the pan.

Arrange a layer of half of the butternut squash. Top with half of the spinach mixture, and then all of the sliced sweet potato.

Drizzle with the cream sauce. Add the remaining half of the spinach, followed by the rest of the butternut squash. Drizzle the rest of the cream sauce over the top.

...m salt, pepper, and nutmeg. Bake for 50-60 minutes until browned. Allow to

Egg Bok Choy and Basil Stir-Fry

Ingredients:
1 garlic clove, minced
2 organic eggs
2 tablespoons olive oil
1 small onion, finely chopped
1-inch piece fresh ginger, chopped
2 red chiles, thinly sliced crosswise
1 cup thinly sliced bok choy stems
1 cup thinly sliced bok choy greens
handful fresh basil leaves, chopped
juice of 1 lime

Instructions:

In a large bowl mix garlic and ginger.

Heat the olive oil in a wok (or a large nonstick skillet) over medium-high heat.

Once it starts to shimmer add onion and chiles. Stir-fry the onions until they start to brown around the edges, about 2 minutes.

Stir in the bok choy stems and stir-fry for 1 minute.

Add the beaten eggs and cook until it's nearly cooked through about 2 minutes, stirring often.

Stir in bok choy greens, basil and lime juice. And stir-fry for 30 seconds or so, until the greens are wilted. Serve immediately.

121. Skinny Eggie Vegetable Stir Fry

Ingredients:
1 lb of Cubed Butternut Squash
1 lb of Green Beans
3 Baby Bok Choys
1½ lb of Eggplants
3 Garlic Cloves
1 small Yellow Onion
½ teaspoon of low sodium salt
½ teaspoon of Black Pepper
1-2 Tablespoons of coconut oil
3 organic eggs

Instructions:

Peel, core, and cut the butternut squash into 1" cubes.

Snap the ends off the green beans and slice at an angle into 1.5" long pieces.

Chop the bok choy leaves from the stems. Slice the stems into 1" thick pieces. Cut the leaves in half.

Slice the eggplants into 1" thick discs, then quarter the disc into wedges. Slice in half if the eggplant is skinny.

Mince the garlic cloves and slice the onions.

Heat a wok and add the cooking oil.

Add the onions and cook until translucent. About 2 minutes.

Add the garlic and cook for another minute.

Add the squash, beans, low sodium salt, pepper

Add the eggplant and bok choy stalks and cook uncovered for another 7-10 minutes.

Add the bok choy leaves and cook for another few minutes, covered.

Beat the eggs and add them to the stir fry …keep stirring till they are cooked through

Salad

- ...sh lemon juice
- ...walnut oil
- ...m salt and freshly ground pepper
- ...rucola leaves and tender stems (about 6 ounces)
- ...lic powder to taste

Instructions:

Pour the lemon juice into a large bowl. Gradually whisk in the oil. Season with low sodium salt and pepper.

Add the greens, toss until evenly dressed and serve at once. This is delicious, and feel free to add tomatoes or grated carrot and onion slices.

Substitution: Any mild green, such as lamb's lettuce will do.

123. Tasty Spring Salad

Ingredients:
5 cups of any salad greens in season of your choice

Dressing:
125 mL (1/2 cup) olive oil
45 mL (3 tbsp) lemon juice
15 mL (1 tbsp) pure mustard powder
45 mL (3 tbsp) capers, minced (optional)
low sodium salt
pepper

Instructions:
Combine salad greens and any other raw vegetables of choice.

Combine oil, lemon juice and mustard. Mix well.

Add capers, low sodium salt and pepper to taste.

Pour dressing over salad, toss and serve.

124. Spinach and Dandelion Pomegranate Salad

Ingredients:
1 small bunch fresh spinach
12 dandelion leaves
1 cup pomegranate seeds
1/2 cup pecan halves

Instructions:
You may substitute appropriate fresh greens for the dandelion and sorrel leaves.

Wash and destem spinach. Pick and wash sorrel and dandelions.

Coarsely chop dandelion leaves, and tear spinach, then toss dandelion, sorrel and spinach together in a stainless steel bowl.

Put aside in refrigerator to drain and cool.

When drained, pour off excess water, and add pomegranate and pecans. Toss with dressing and serve.

125. Pure Delish Spinach Salad

Ingredients:
2 bunches fresh spinach
1 bunch scallions, chopped
juice of 1 lemon
1/4 tbsp olive oil
pepper to taste

optional: rice vinegar to taste

Instructions:
Wash spinach well. Drain and chop.

After a few minutes, squeeze excess water.

Add scallions, lemon juice, oil and pepper.

126. Sexy Salsa Salad

Ingredients:
1 bunch of cilantro
5-6 roma tomatoes
1 small yellow or red onion
1 small chili pepper
2 ripe avocados.
handful of rucola leaf

Instructions:
Chop cilantro, dice tomatoes, dice onion, finely dice chili pepper, dice avocado.

After dicing each ingredient add to large bowl. Add rucola to bowl.

When finished, toss.

127. Eastern Avo Salad

Ingredients:
2 to 3 lbs. of tomatoes
4 med. or lg. avocados (or 1lb chopped or ground nuts or seeds)
4 stalks celery
4 lg. red (or green) bell peppers
2 lbs. bok choy stalks and greens

Instructions:
Dice the tomatoes, celery and the bell peppers.

Quarter, peel and dice the avocados.

Cut up the bok choy.

Place all ingredients in a bowl and mix together.

128. Curry Coconut Salad

Ingredients:
6 large ripe tomatoes, peeled, seeded and chopped
1 small white onion, grated
1/4 tsp. coarsely ground pepper
1/2 cup coconut cream
2 Tbsp minced fresh parsley
1 tsp. curry powder

Instructions:
Combine tomatoes, onion and pepper; cover and chill for 3 hours.

Combine coconut cream, parsley and curry; cover and chill for 3 hours.

To serve, spoon tomato mixture into small bowls and top each with a spoonful of coconut cream mixture.

129. Jalapeno Salsa

Ingredients:
1 jalapeno pepper seeded and chopped fine
2 large ripe tomatoes, peeled and chopped
1 medium onion, minced
2 tbsp olive oil
juice of 1 lemon
1/2 tsp dried oregano
pepper to taste

Instructions:
Combine all ingredients and mix well. Refrigerate covered until ready to eat.

130. Beet Sprout Divine Salad

Ingredients:
1/2 pound Brussels sprouts, ends trimmed, outer leaves removed, and cut in half lengthwise
4 small red beets, tops trimmed to 1/2-inch, washed and cut in half lengthwise
4 tablespoons plus 1/3 cup extra virgin olive oil
1 tablespoon paleo Dijon mustard
Stevia to taste
Squeeze of lemon juice
Coarse low sodium salt
Grinding coarse black pepper
1 small red onion thinly sliced into rings

Instructions:
Preheat the oven to 350.

Pour 2 tablespoons olive oil in a baking dish. Toss the Brussels sprouts in the oil; sprinkle them with low sodium salt and pepper and roast them for 20 minutes.

Turn them once during the cooking. They are done when a small knife easily pierces them.

Pour 2 tablespoons of the olive oil on a sheet of aluminum foil and place

it on a baking sheet. Toss the beet halves in the olive oil. Sprinkle them with low sodium salt and pepper and, keeping them in a single layer, fold and seal the foil over them. Bake on the baking sheet until a knife easily pierces them.

When cool enough to handle, peel the beets and cut them into 1/4-inch slices.

Meanwhile combine the 1/3 cup olive oil, mustard, stevia, lemon juice and low sodium salt and pepper in a small bowl.

Toss the Ingredients, add the dressing and serve at room temperature.

131. Divine Carrot Salad

Ingredients:
3 tablespoons fresh lemon juice
1 tablespoon Olive oil
1 pressed garlic clove
1-1/2 pound carrots, peeled and rectangle and lightly steamed

Instructions:
Mix dressing ingredients in a small bowl. Add carrots; toss to mix.

Let stand at room temperature for one hour and then serve.

132. Cauliflower Couscous

Ingredients:
1 1/2 Lbs cauliflower florets
1/2 cup parsley (VERY finely chopped)
1/2 cup fresh mint (very FINELY chopped)
1/2 cup chopped red onion
One cucumber finely cubed
4.5 to 5 Tbls fresh lime juice (about 2 fruits)
2 Tbls olive oil
1 teas low sodium salt
1 teas black pepper

Instructions:
In a food processor (NOT A BLENDER) pulse cauliflower until it looks like rice. Set aside in serving bowl.

In food processor- blend parsley, mint, onion, lime juice, olive oil, and low sodium salt and pepper into a smooth paste.

Pour over cauliflower and cucumber and blend well.

133. Mouthwatering Mushroom Salad

Ingredients:
2/3 cup olive oil
1/3 cup fresh lemon juice
One tablespoon red wine vinegar
1 tsp dried thyme
pepper and garlic powder to taste
1 pound fresh mushrooms, thinly sliced
1/4 cup minced parsley
Rucola leaves

Instructions:
Combine all ingredients except the mushrooms, parsley and greens, and mix well.

Add the mushrooms and toss with 2 forks. Cover and let stand at room temperature.

At serving time, drain and sprinkle with the parsley. Pile in a serving dish lined with greens.

134. Skinny Sweet Potato Salad

Ingredients:
4 small sweet potatoes
1 tablespoon olive oil extra virgin
1 teaspoon mustard powder
4 celery stalks, sliced 1/4-inch thick
1 small red bell pepper, cut into 1/4-inch dice
2 scallions, finely chopped
low sodium salt and pepper
1/2 cup coarsely chopped toasted pecans
Chopped fresh chives

Instructions:
Preheat oven to 400°F.

Wrap each sweet potato in foil and bake for 1 hour.

Unwrap; let cool. Peel; cut into 3/4-inch chunks.

In a large bowl, mix oil and mustard. Add sweet potatoes, celery,

red pepper and scallions; toss gently.

Season to taste with low sodium salt and pepper.

Cover and refrigerate about 1 hour.

Fold in pecans and sprinkle with chives.

135. Fabulous Brownie Treats

Ingredients:
1 1/2 cups walnuts
Pinch of low sodium salt
1 tsp vanilla
1/3 cup unsweetened cocoa powder
Stevia to taste

Instructions:
Add walnuts and low sodium salt to a blender or food processor. Mix until the walnuts are finely ground.

Add the vanilla, and cocoa powder etc to the blender. Mix well until everything is combined.

With the blender still running, add a couple drops of water at a time to make the mixture stick together.

Using a spatula, transfer the mixture into a bowl. Using your hands, form small round balls, rolling in your palm.

136. Rose Banana Delicious Brownies

Ingredients:
2 red beets, cooked
2 bananas
2 eggs
1/2 cup unsweetened cacao powder
1/3 cup almond flour
1 tsp baking powder
3 tablespoons crushes mixed nuts
Stevia to taste

Instructions:
Combine all ingredients in a food processor, and blend until smooth.

Stir in the nut bits

Pour into a well-greased pan about 8x8 inches

Bake at 325 for about 40 minutes.

137. Pristine Pumpkin Divine

Ingredients:
2 cups blanched almond flour
½ cup flaxseed meal
2 teaspoons ground cinnamon (optional)
Stevia to taste
½ teaspoon low sodium salt
1 egg
1 cup pumpkin puree
1 tablespoon vanilla extract

Instructions:
Mix together the almond flour, flaxseed meal, cinnamon, and low sodium salt

In a separate bowl, whisk the egg, pumpkin and vanilla extract using a rubber spatula.

Gently mix dry and wet ingredients to form a batter being careful not to over mix or the batter will get oily and dense.

Spoon the batter onto a 9-inch pan lined with parchment paper or grease the pan

bake at 350°F until a toothpick inserted into the center comes out clean, approximately 25 minutes.

138. Secret Brownies

Ingredients:
1 c. raw almonds
1/2 c. raw cashews
4-5 Tbs. cocoa powder
1 Tbs. cashew butter
Stevia to taste

Instructions:
Combine all ingredients in the food processor.

Whir until somewhat smooth.

Press into 8×8" glass baking dish.

Chill until ready to serve.

139. Spectacular Spinach Brownies

Ingredients:
1 ¼ cups frozen chopped spinach
6 oz sugar free chocolate
½ cup extra virgin coconut oil
½ cup coconut oil
6 eggs
Stevia to taste
½ cup cocoa powder
1 Tspn vanilla pod
¼ tsp baking soda
½ tsp low sodium salt
½ tsp cream of tartar
pinch cinnamon

Instructions:

Preheat oven to 325F. Line a 9"x13" baking pan with wax paper or use a silicone baking pan.

Melt coconut oil and chocolate together over low heat on the stove top or medium power in the microwave. Add vanilla and stir to incorporate. Let cool.

Mix cocoa powder, baking soda, cream of tartar, low sodium salt and cinnamon.

Blend spinach, egg, together in a food processor or blender, until completely smooth (2-4 minutes).

Add coconut oil to food processor and process until full incorporated.

Add melted chocolate mixture and 3 or 4 drops stevia liquid to egg mixture slowly and processing/blending constantly.

Mix in dry ingredients and process/stir to fully incorporate.

Pour batter into prepared baking pan and spread out with a spatula.

Bake for 40 minutes. Cool completely in pan. Cut into squares. Enjoy!

140. Choco-coco Brownies

Ingredients:
6 Tablespoons of coconut oil
6 ounces of Sugar free Chocolate
4 Tablespoons of Packed Coconut Flour (20g)
¼ cup of Unsweetened Cocoa Powder (30g)
2 Eggs
½ teaspoon of Baking Soda
¼ teaspoon of low sodium salt
Extra coconut oil for pan greasing
Stevia to taste

Instructions:
Preheat the oven to 350F. Grease an 8x8 baking pan and line with parchment paper.

Ensure eggs are at room temperature. You may run them under warm water for about 10 seconds while shelled.

Gently melt the semisweet chocolate and oil in a double boiler. You may use the microwave at 50% heat at 30 second intervals with intermittent stirring.

Stir in unsweetened cocoa powder.

Sift together the superfine coconut flour, baking soda, stevia and low sodium salt.

Beat the eggs and add the dry ingredients. Beat until combined

Add the rest of the wet ingredients and beat until incorporated.

Pour the batter into the lined 8x8 pan.

Bake for 25-30 minutes at 350F until a toothpick inserted into the center of the batter comes out clean.

When done, remove from the oven and let cool in the pan for at least 15 minutes.

141. Coco – Walnut Brownie Bites

Ingredients:
2/3 cup raw walnut halves and pieces
1/3 cup unsweetened cocoa powder
1 tablespoon vanilla extract
1 to 2 tablespoons coconut milk
2/3 cups shredded unsweetened coconut

Instructions:

Pulse coconut in food processor for 30 seconds to a minute to form coconut crumbs. Remove from food processor and set aside.

Add unsweetened cocoa powder and walnuts to food processor, blend until walnuts become fine crumbs, but do not over process or you will get some kind of chocolate walnut butter.

Place in the food processor the cocoa walnut crumbs. Add vanilla. Process until mixture starts to combine.

Add coconut milk. You will know the consistency is right when the dough combines into a ball in the middle of the food processor.

If dough is too runny add a tablespoon or more cocoa powder to bring it back to a dough like state.

Transfer dough to a bowl and cover with plastic wrap. Refrigerate for at least 2 hours. Cold dough is much easier to work with. I left my dough in the fridge over night. You could put it in the freezer if you need to speed the process up.

Roll the dough balls in coconut crumbs, pressing the crumbs gently into the ball. Continue until all dough is gone.

142. Best Ever Banana Surprise Cake

Ingredients:

Bottom Fruit Layer:
2 tbsps coconut oil, melted
1 small banana, sliced, or ¼ cup blueberries for low carb version
2 tbsps walnut pieces * optional, can omit for nut free.
Stevia to taste
1 tsp ground cinnamon.

Top Cake Layer:
2 eggs, beaten.
Stevia to taste
¼ cup unsweetened coconut milk, or unsweetened almond milk.
1 tsp organic GF vanilla extract, or 1 tsp ground vanilla bean
½ tsp baking soda.
1 tsp apple cider vinegar.
1 small banana, mashed, or ¼ cup blueberries for lower carb version.
⅓ cup coconut flour

Instructions:

Preheat oven to 350 F, and lightly grease a 9 inch cake pan.

Place 2 tbsps coconut oil into cake pan, and put pan into preheating oven for a couple minutes to melt butter or oil. Once melted, make sure butter or oil is evenly distributed all over the bottom of the pan.

Sprinkle 2-4 drops stevia sweetener all over the melted oil.

Sprinkle 1 tsp cinnamon on top of sweetener layer.

Layer banana slices or blueberries on top of butter- sweetener layer, as seen in photo above. Add optional walnut pieces to fruit layer. Set aside.

In a large mixing bowl combine all the "top cake layer" ingredients except for the coconut flour. Mix thoroughly, then add the coconut flour and mix well, scraping sides of bowl, and braking up any coconut flour clumps.
Spoon cake batter on top of fruit layer in cake pan
Spread cake batter evenly across entire pan.
Bake for 25 minutes or until top of cake is browned and center is set.
Remove from oven and let cool completely.
Use a butter knife between cake and edge of pan and slide around to loosen cake from pan. Turn cake pan upside down onto a large plate or serving platter.
Slice and serve.
Should be stored in fridge, if serving later.

Paleo Diet Recipes 365 Days Of Anti-Inflammatory Recipes
By Mercedes Del Rey

143. Choco Cookie Delight

Ingredients:
1/2 cup dark chocolate sugar free chips
1/2 cup coconut milk (thick fat from top of can)
2 eggs
1 cup almond flour
pinch of low sodium salt
1/2 teaspoon vanilla extract
1/4 teaspoon baking powder

Vanilla glaze:
1/2 cup coconut butter, liquid
Stevia to taste
1 /2 teaspoon vanilla extract

Chocolate Glaze:
1/2 cup chocolate chips
Stevia powder for decoration

Instructions:
Place a small sauce pan over low heat and melt your chocolate and coconut milk together (only keep the heat on long enough to melt them together)

While melting, place your 2 eggs in a stand mixer with the whisk, or use a hand mixer with the whisk and beat your eggs until they are fluffy, about 1 minute

Add your coconut milk and chocolate to your eggs and mix well

Stir in your almond flour, low sodium salt, vanilla extract and baking powder

Mix well ensuring everything is combined

Pipe your batter into the cookie wells ensuring you fill higher than the halfway point

Remove from the cookie maker, gently insert the sticks and place everything in the freezer for 30-45 minutes

Vanilla Glaze:

Combine your coconut butter, stevia, and vanilla extract in a small glass to make it easy to dip

You can keep this glass in hot water to keep the glaze more liquidy to make the dipping easier

Chocolate Glaze:

Melt your chocolate chips over a double boiler and keep the heat low and them liquid – then spread over cooled cookies!

144. Choco Triple Delight

Ingredients:
Cake:
1 cup almond flour (or 3 oz ground raw pumpkin seeds for nut-free version)
3 tbsp Raw Cacao Powder
1 tbsp coconut flour
1 tsp baking powder
1/2 tsp baking soda
1/8th tsp Stevia
3 tbsp melted Raw Cacao Butter or coconut oil)
Pinch of low sodium salt
1 large pastured egg
2 tbsp coconut milk (or dairy of choice)
1 tsp pure vanilla extract
2 oz 80% cocoa bar, chopped
Top with 2 tbsp chopped nut of choice,
Optional: 1/8th tsp low sodium salt sprinkled on top of cake before baking

Chocolate Drizzle:
2 tbsp coconut cream concentrate, warmed
3 tbsp water (or coconut milk)
3 tbsp Cacao powder
1/2 tbsp pure vanilla extract
Stevia to taste

Instructions:
Preheat oven to 350 degrees F.

Oil the sides and bottom of 8 inch cake pan.

Line the bottom of the pan with parchment paper and set aside.

In a medium bowl, add dry ingredients. Use a sifter to insure that all ingredients are blended well and that there are no lumps.

Add remaining ingredients (except nuts and optional salt) to dry ingredients and mix. Taste for sweetness and adjust if necessary.

Press (or spread with angled spatula) into a 8 inch cake pan. Sprinkle with nuts. Bake for 11-14 minutes.

DO NOT OVER BAKE! Remove from oven and serve warm or allow to cool and top with Chocolate Drizzle.

Chocolate Drizzle:

In a small bowl, blend coconut cream concentrate and water until smooth.

Add cacao powder, vanilla and stevia. Whisk until creamy.

Taste for sweetness and adjust if necessary. Drizzle over the cake.

145. Peach and Almond Cake

Ingredients:
2 whole peaches
300g almond meal
6 eggs
Stevia to taste
1 tsp baking soda

Instructions:
Cover the peaches in water in a saucepan and boil for about 2 hours.

Preheat the oven to 180 degrees Celsius and line the bottom of a 24cm pan with baking paper.

Lightly beat the eggs.

Blend the eggs and peaches (quarter them first) thoroughly in a food processor.

Add the rest of the ingredients to the food processor, again blending thoroughly.

Pour mixture into the lined tin and bake for roughly an hour.

146. Apple Cinnamon Walnut Bonanza

Ingredients:
For the cake:
1 cup almond flour
2 tablespoons coconut flour
Stevia to taste
1 tablespoon cinnamon
1 teaspoon baking soda
1/4 teaspoon low sodium salt
1 tablespoon coconut butter, plus more for greasing the pan
2 eggs
1/2 cup cream from a can of refrigerated coconut milk
1 teaspoon vanilla
1 cup grated apple (about 1 large apple)
For the topping:
1 1/2 cups walnuts (or pecans, if you prefer)
1/2 cup almond flour
4 tablespoons melted coconut butter
Stevia to taste
1 tablespoon cinnamon
pinch low sodium salt

Instructions:
Preheat your oven to 350° and grease a 8 x 8 baking dish.

Make the topping: pulse the walnuts in a food processor 10-12 times or until they are course crumbs. Add the remaining ingredients and pulse 2-3 more times until combined. Set aside.

Wipe out and dry the bowl of your food processor and add your dry **cake** ingredients. (almond flour through low sodium salt) Pulse a few times to mix.

Cut the tablespoon of butter into smaller chunks and add it to the dry ingredients. Pulse 8-10 times or until it's cut in to the dry ingredients, similar to if you were making a pie crust.

In a small bowl, mix your wet cake ingredients (eggs through vanilla) and whisk until well combined. Stir in grated apple.

Add to the food processor and mix until combined. Scrape down the sides once or twice to make sure it's well mixed.

Pour into the prepared baking dish and sprinkle the topping over, as evenly as you can.

Bake for 30-35 minutes, or until a toothpick inserted into the center comes out clean.

Allow to cool, and enjoy!

147. Chestnut- Cacao Cake

Ingredients:
100g (1 cup + 1 heaping tablespoon) chestnut flour
50g (1/2 cup) ground almonds (almond flour)
3 eggs, separate
1/2 teaspoon cream of tartar
35g (1/2 cup) raw cacao powder
Stevia to taste
3/4 cup coconut milk
1/2 teaspoon baking soda
Crushed chesnuts

Instructions:
Preheat oven to 180C fan (350F).

Grease a pie/tart pan.

In a clean mixing bowl, beat the egg whites and cream of tartar until stiff peaks form. Set aside.

In another mixing bowl, cream the egg yolks, chestnut flour, ground almonds, stevia, raw cacao, baking soda and coconut milk.

Fold in the egg whites and blend until the white is no longer showing.

Pour into the pie/tart mold.

Sprinkle with crushed chestnuts, if desired.

Bake for 35-40 minutes on the middle rack.

148. Extra Dark Choco Delight

Ingredients:
1 egg
½ very ripe avocado
¼ cup full fat canned coconut milk
2 tbsp cacao powder
1 tbsp carob powder
pinch low sodium salt
pinch cinnamon
1 scoop vanilla flavored hemp protein powder
10g raw hazelnuts
2 tbsp unsweetened shredded coconut
Stevia to taste

Instructions:
Add the egg, avocado and coconut milk to a small food processor and process until very smooth and process until very smooth and creamy.

Add cacao powder, carob powder, low sodium salt, cinnamon and protein powder and process again until well combined and creamy.

Add hazelnuts and shredded coconut and give a few extra spins until the hazelnuts are reduced to tiny little pieces.

Serve immediately or refrigerate until ready to serve.

Garnish with a little dollop of coconut cream and cacao nibs or shredded coconut and crushed hazelnuts.

This will keep in the refrigerator for a few days in an airtight container.

149. Nut Butter Truffles

Ingredients:
5 tablespoons sunflower seed butter
1 tablespoon coconut oil
2 teaspoons vanilla extract
¾ cup almond flour
1 tablespoon flaxseed meal
pinch of low sodium salt
¼ cup sugar free dark chocolate chips
1 tablespoon cacao butter
chopped almonds (optional)
stevia to taste

Instructions:
Add sunflower seed butter, coconut oil, vanilla, almond flour, flaxseed meal and low sodium salt to a large bowl. Please note that you may find a thin layer of oil in the sunflower seed butter jar that separates from the butter and rises to the top. Be sure to mix oil and butter together before scooping into bowl.

Using your hands mix until all ingredients are incorporated (I like using gloves when mixing so the oils from my skin do not get into the mixture)

Roll the dough into 1-inch balls and place them on a sheet of parchment paper and refrigerate for 30 minutes (using 2 teaspoons for each truffle will yield about 14 truffles)

Melt the chocolate chips in a double boiler along with the cacao butter

Dip each truffle in the melted chocolate, one at the time, and place them back on the pan with parchment paper

Top with chopped almonds and refrigerate until the chocolate is firm

150. Fetching Fudge

Ingredients:
1 cup coconut butter
1/4 cup coconut oil
1/4 cup cocoa
1/4 cup cocoa powder + 1 Tbsp
Stevia to taste
1 tsp vanilla

Instructions:
In the pot, gently melt the cocoa butter on low (number 2)

When it is half melted add the butter, the coconut oil and the coconut spread and gently mix with the whisk as it melts

Add vanilla, and stevia and whisk in well

Add the cocoa powder and whisk in well

Be sure to take the pot off the heat when the fat is melted and keep whisking until it is smooth and all the lumps are out — you don't want to overheat this

Pour into the 8 x 8 pan that is lined with parchment paper

Refrigerate for 1 – 2 hours

When solid, pull the parchment paper out of the pan, put the block of fudge on a flat surface and cut into small squares

Enjoy! This will melt rather quickly — but it won't last long!

151. Choco – Almond Delights

Ingredients:
1 c. toasted hazelnuts
1 c. raw almonds
2/3 c. raw almond butter
5 Tbs. raw cacao powder (or unsweetened cocoa powder)
1/2 tsp. vanilla extract
1/4 c. unsweetened, shredded coconut
Stevia to taste

Instructions:
Combine all the ingredients, except for the coconut, in the food processor. Whir until smooth. This will take a few minutes and may require scraping down the sides of the bowl one or more times.

Line a mini muffin tin with plastic wrap. Spoon dollops of the sweet mixture into the lined tin cups and form into "mounds." Freeze until well formed. Remove mounds from plastic and tin and flip for presentation. Sprinkle with shredded coconut.

152. Chococups

Ingredients:
4 eggs
Stevia to taste
1/3 cup coconut flour
1/4 cup cacao powder
1/2 teaspoon baking soda
1/4 cup coconut oil (melted in microwave)
1/4 cup cacao butter (melted in microwave)

For topping:
1 can coconut cream (chilled in fridge overnight)
Cacao nibs to decorate.

Instructions:
Heat oven to 170 degrees Celsius (338F)

Grease 10 muffin pans with coconut oil.

Beat eggs with electric beaters.

Add coconut flour, baking soda and cacao powder.

Beat well and add stevia

Add melted coconut oil, cacao butter and mix.

Spoon mixture into 10 greased muffin pans.

Bake for 12-15 minutes until risen and top springs back.

Cool in pans.

Beat the solid coconut cream with electric beaters until creamy. Add honey to taste if you wish.

Pipe coconut cream onto top of cakes.

153. Choco Coco Cookies

Ingredients:
Stevia powder – 1 teaspoon – or to taste
1 cup coconut flour
½ cup coconut oil
½ cup coconut milk, (from the can)
2 Teaspoons vanilla extract
¼ Teaspoon low sodium salt
2½ cups finely shredded coconut
1 cup big flake coconut
⅔ cup dark sugar free chocolate chunks or chocolate chips (I used 80% dark chocolate)
Optional: ½ cup almond or cashew butter

Instructions:
In a large saucepan, combine the, coconut oil, and coconut milk. Bring the mixture to a boil, and boil for 2-3 minutes.

Remove from the heat and add the vanilla, low sodium salt, and coconut flour and coconut. Stir to combine. If you're using the almond or cashew butter, mix it in thoroughly. Finally, add the chocolate chunks and combine, stirring as little as possible to keep the chunks intact.

Portion the cookie on a parchment lined baking sheet and let cool. This version of no-bakes takes a full 3-4 hours to fully set up, but you don't have to wait that long because they're really good warm and gooey.

154. Apple Spice Spectacular

Ingredients:
1 cup unsweetened almond butter
Stevia to taste
1 egg
1 tsp baking soda
1/2 tsp low sodium salt
half an apple, diced 1 tsp cinnamon
1/4 tsp ground cloves
1/8 tsp nutmeg
1 tsp fresh ginger, grated on a microplane

Instructions:
Pre-heat oven to 350 degress F.

In a large bowl, combine almond butter, stevia, egg, baking soda, and low sodium salt until well incorporated. Add apple, spices, and ginger and stir to combine.

Spoon batter onto a baking sheet (you may have to spread the batter a little to get it into a round shape) about 1-2 inches apart from each other--they'll spread a bit.

Bake about 10 minutes, or until slightly set.

Remove cookies and allow to cool on pan for about 5-10 minutes. Then finish cooling on a cooling rack.

155. Absolute Almond Bites

Ingredients:
1 1/2 cups almond flour
1/4 teaspoon low sodium salt
1/4 teaspoon baking soda (gluten-free, if necessary)
1/8 teaspoon cinnamon
2 tablespoons melted coconut oil
Stevia to taste
1 1/4 teaspoon vanilla extract
1/4 teaspoon almond extract or almond flavoring
12 to 15 whole almonds; sprouted or soaked and dehydrated

Instructions:

Preheat oven to 325°F. Line a baking sheet with parchment paper.

In a medium bowl combine almond flour, low sodium salt, baking soda, and cinnamon. Mix well, breaking up any lumps.

In a small bowl, place coconut oil, vanilla, almond extract or flavoring. Whisk until well combined.

Add wet ingredients to dry ingredients and stir until combined…add stevia

Roll level-tablespoon-sized (using a measuring spoon) portions of dough into balls and place on baking sheet. Flatten slightly with the heel of your hand and press one almond into the center of each cookie.

Bake 15 to 17 minutes or until light golden brown. Allow to cool on baking sheet for a few minutes before transferring to cooling rack.

Store in an airtight container. Can be frozen.

156. Eastern Spice Delights

Ingredients:
1 3/4 cups + 4 tbsp almond meal
1/8 tsp low sodium salt
3/4 tsp ground ginger
3/4 tsp cinnamon
1/4 tsp ground cloves
1/4 tsp cardamom
1/8 tsp nutmeg
1/2 cup coconut oil (in solid form)
Stevia to taste
1 tsp vanilla extract

Instructions:
Preheat oven to 350F.

Combine all the dry ingredients in a large bowl. In a small bowl, mix together the oil, maple syrup, and vanilla until completely blended. Pour the wet ingredients over the dry ingredients and mix well.

Drop the cookie dough on a cookie sheet. It will spread a bit as it cooks (and thus flatten), but not an awful lot.

Bake for 10-12 minutes. These cookies will not look golden when they're done. Makes two dozens.

157. Berry Ice Cream and Almond Delight

Ingredients:

For the Ice Cream:
1 can full fat coconut milk
Stevia to taste
2 tbsp vanilla
1 cup fresh strawberries, cut into fourths

For the crisp:
1/3 cup almond flour
3 tbsp sunflower seed butter (or almond butter)
1/2 tsp vanilla
1 tbsp honey
low sodium salt to taste

Instructions:

For the ice cream:

Combine coconut milk and vanilla together in a small saucepan over medium heat and stir until ingredients are well combined (just a few minutes).

Transfer milk mixture to a small bowl and place in the freezer for two hours.

Next, add strawberries to a small saucepan and bring to a low boil.

Turn heat to medium-low and allow to cook until they start breaking down into a sauce-like mixture, leaving small chunks.

Place strawberries in refrigerator while the ice cream hardens.

For the crisp:

Combine all ingredients and mix until you get a "crumble" consistency.

Place crisp in refrigerator until ready to use.

After two hours, place milk mixture into your ice cream maker along with the strawberries and use as directed.

When ice cream is ready, scoop and serve with crisp sprinkled on top.

158. Creamy Caramely Ice Cream

Ingredients:
Delicious Instant Caramel Topping:
2 heaped tablespoons of hulled tahini
Stevia to taste
2 tablespoons of coconut milk
1/2 teaspoon of vanilla

Delicious Instant Ice Cream:
4 frozen bananas, chopped
4 tablespoons coconut milk
1 teaspoon of vanilla

Instructions:
Spoon the tahini and stevia into a cup and stir with a fork to combine. Mix in the coconut milk and vanilla. Refrain from eating it while you make your ice cream.

Place the ingredients into food processor or blender, blend until the mixture is an ice cream consistency.

Spoon the ice cream into bowls, drizzle generously with the caramel topping, sprinkle with low sodium salt if you desire. Enjoy!

159. Cheeky Cherry Ice

Ingredients:
14oz. cans 365 Coconut Milk (Full Fat)
Stevia to taste
1 ½ tsp. vanilla extract
2 cups fresh cherries, pitted and diced

Instructions:
In a large bowl, combine coconut milk, stevia and vanilla and stir well.

Chill for 1-2 hours.

Transfer to ice-cream maker and process according to manufacturer directions.

Add diced cherries to the mixture during the last 5-10 minutes of processing.

160. Choco - Coconut Berry Ice

Ingredients:
Follow recipe of berry ice cream and almond delight for the ice cream only
4 ounces sugar free dark chocolate - 75% cacao content
¼ cup coconut milk
2 cups fresh berries (I used raspberries)
Stevia to taste

Instructions:
Make the Homemade Coconut Ice Cream,

While the ice cream is freezing in the machine, break the chocolate into pieces and place in a small saucepan.

Add the coconut milk and melt the two together, stirring over low heat.

When the chocolate mixture is completely smooth, pour the chocolate over the ice cream and stir to create 'ripples'. If your ice cream if thoroughly frozen, soften in the fridge for 20 minutes before stirring in the chocolate.

Serve immediately with the fresh berries, or freeze for an additional 3-4 hours for a firmer texture.

161. Creamy Berrie Pie

Ingredients:
Crust:
3 cups almonds
½ Teaspoon cinnamon
½ cup honey
2 Tablespoons coconut oil
1 Tablespoon lemon zest
1 Teaspoon almond extract
pinch of low sodium salt

Filling:
2 Teaspoons plant-based gelatin, dissolved in 2 Tablespoons hot water
⅓ cup freshly squeezed lemon juice
Stevia to taste
1 can coconut milk, chilled
4 cups blueberries for serving

Instructions:
Place the almonds and cinnamon in a food processor and pulse until your desired texture is reached. I like to leave some bigger pieces for texture. Add the rest of the crust ingredients and pulse until a sticky dough forms. Pat the crust into a pie plate, (use water to keep your hands from sticking to the crust).

For the filling, mix the gelatin and water together. Stir to dissolve and immediately add the lemon juice. If the gelatin gets clumpy, place the mixture over hot water until it melts again. Pour the coconut milk into an electric mixer, add the stevia and whip on high until peaks form, about 15 minutes. Add the gelatin mixture to the whipped cream. Pour the filling into the crust. The filling will seem thin, but don't worry it will set up in the refrigerator.

Chill for at least 4 hours until set, and serve with lots of berries!

162. Peachy Creamy Peaches

Ingredients:
3 medium ripe peaches, cut in half with pit removed
1 tsp vanilla
1 can coconut milk, refrigerated
1/4 cup chopped walnuts
Cinnamon and stevia (to taste)

Instructions:
Place peaches on the grill with the cut side down first. Grill on medium-low heat until soft, about 3-5 minutes on each side.

Scoop cream off the top of the can of chilled coconut milk. Whip together coconut cream and vanilla with handheld mixer. Drizzle over each peach. Top with cinnamon and chopped walnuts to garnish.

163. Spiced Apple Bake

Ingredients:
2 apples of your choice
1/4 cup walnuts
1/4 tablespoon nutmeg
1/4 tablespoon cinnamon
1/4 tablespoon ground cloves

Instructions:
Preheat oven to 350 degrees Fahrenheit.

Slice the very top and very bottom off of each apple. (The top allows for more room to stuff with goodies, the bottom allows the apples to soak up all the nice sauce).

Core both apples to the bottom, but not all the way through.

Mix spices, walnuts, and raisins in a small bowl.

Pour half of the spice mixture into each apple.

Place on baking sheet and bake 20-25 minutes, or until apples are soft. I like to pour any remaining sauce mixture into the bottom of the pan so the apples can soak up the flavors.

164. Sexy Dessert Pan

Ingredients:
Crust:
1 1/2 cups pecans
3/4 cup dates
4 tbsp coconut oil

Second Layer:
2/3 cup cashew butter
1/3 cup palm shortening
2 tsp apple cider vinegar
1/2 tsp lemon juice
Pinch low sodium salt

Third Layer:
1 cup coconut flour
1 cup coconut milk
Stevia to taste
1 tsp vanilla extract

Fourth Layer:
1/2 cup coconut milk
1/2 cup coconut butter
1/2 cup cacao powder
2 tbsp honey

Fifth Layer:
1/2 cup coconut butter
1/4 cup coconut milk
Stevia to taste

Sixth Layer:
Grated dark sugar free chocolate, at least 80% cacao

Instructions:
To make the crust, roughly chop the pecans then pit and chop the dates. Load both into a food processor and pulse until ground but still crumbly. Transfer to a bowl and work in the coconut oil, then press the sticky mixture into a single smooth layer at the bottom of a square 8x8 cake pan.

Transfer to the refrigerator to chill while you begin the second layer. To make the second layer, combine its ingredients very well in a medium mixing bowl. Spoon over the chilled crust, smoothing as much as possible with the back of a spoon. Place the pan back in the fridge.

To make the third layer, mix its ingredients together in a mixing bowl and then spoon over the chilled, hardened second layer. Smooth as much as possible, then chill.

Add the fourth layer by combining its ingredients and then layering it into the pan in the same way as the previous layers.

For the fifth layer, mix the coconut shortening, coconut milk and stevia with a hand mixer until very smooth and spoon over the chilled fourth layer.

Before placing the pan back into the refrigerator after adding the fifth layer, grate very dark chocolate over the top to the depth of your preference. Chill the pan for an additional half hour or more, then slice with a sharp knife and serve.

165. Pretty Pumpkin Delights

Ingredients:
For Crust:
1 cup hazelnuts (preferably soaked and dehydrated for better digestion)
1/2 cup raw pumpkin seeds (preferably soaked and dehydrated for better
1 TBS coconut oil
2 pinches of low sodium salt
Stevia to taste

For Filling:
1 cup cooked pumpkin puree
1/2 cup coconut
2 TBS coconut oil
Stevia to taste
1/2 tsp vanilla extract
1/4 tsp cinnamon powder
1/4 tsp ginger powder
1/8 tsp allspice
1/8 tsp clove powder

For Chocolate Drizzle:
2 TBS coconut butter
2 TBS coconut oil
2 TBS raw cacao (or unsweetened cocoa)
Stevia to taste
a pinch or 2 of low sodium salt

Instructions:
To Make the crust: Line mini muffin tins with unbleached mini paper liners. Process all crust ingredients in a food processor until well combined and resembles a coarse flour. Spoon 1 and 1/2 tsp of mixture into each of the 24 mini cups. Use your thumb to press down mixture firmly to create a solid bottom layer for these cute little yummies. Place in freezer to harden.

To make filling: Melt coconut butter and coconut oil in a double boiler. Remove from heat and add rest of filling ingredients. Go ahead and mix it up real good here until creamy smooth. Remove crusts from freezer and spoon about 3/4 TBS of filling over your prepared crusts. Return to freezer to harden, at least 2 hours.

To make chocolate drizzle: Once mini bites have hardened, gently melt coconut butter and coconut oil in a double boiler. Remove from heat and add rest of drizzle ingredients. Allow to cool slightly to thicken. Pour into small plastic bag, cut a TINY hole in the corner, and drizzle over treats in any fashion that you want.

Now it's time to enjoy these amazing delights. Store leftovers in freezer as they are best cold. (That is, if there are any leftovers. Ours got dusted off in one day.)

Paleo Diet Recipes 365 Days Of Anti-Inflammatory Recipes
By Mercedes Del Rey

166. Macadamia Pineapple Bonanza

Ingredients:
Crust:
½ cup almond flour
4 tablespoons raw cacao powder
⅓ cup macadamia nuts
½ teaspoon vanilla extract
Stevia to taste
1½ teaspoons coconut oil, melted
Filling:
2 eggs
1 cup fresh pineapple, chopped
1⅓ cup shredded coconut, unsweetened
1 tablespoon fresh lime juice
1 tablespoon vanilla extract
Stevia to taste
½ cup almond flour
pinch of low sodium salt

Instructions:
Crust:

In a large bowl, mix the almond flour and cacao powder.

Chop the macadamia nuts in a food processor and add it to the bowl.

Add vanilla extract and coconut oil to the dry mixture and using your hands, mix to combine ingredients.

Spread the mixture evenly on the bottom of an 8x8-inch pan lined with parchment paper. Be sure to use one large piece of paper covering the entire pan that overlaps on all four sides

Filing:

In a large bowl beat the 2 eggs

Mix in the pineapple, 1 cup of shredded coconut (reserve the remaining ⅓ cup for the top), lime juice, vanilla and stevia.

Gently mix in the almond flour and low sodium salt with rubber spatula.

Pour mixture over the crust and sprinkle top with remaining shredded coconut.

Bake at 350°F for approximately 20 minutes or until the top starts to brown and the pineapple/coconut layer is firm.

Set pan on a wire rack and allow it to cool before cutting into squares. Store in the refrigerator.

Paleo Diet Recipes 365 Days Of Anti-Inflammatory Recipes
By Mercedes Del Rey

167. Lemony Lemon Delights

Ingredients:
Crust:
1 cup almond flour
1/4 cup almond butter
Stevia to taste
1 tbsp coconut butter
1 tsp vanilla
1/2 tsp baking powder
1/4 tsp low sodium salt

Filling:
3 eggs
Stevia to taste
1/4 cup lemon juice
2 1/2 tbsp coconut flour
1 tbsp lemon zest, finely grated
Pinch of low sodium salt

Instructions:
Preheat oven to 350.

Coat 9×9 baking dish with coconut oil or butter.

Combine all crust ingredients in food processor until a "crumble" forms.

Press crust evenly into the bottom of pan.

Using a fork, prick a few holes into crust.

Bake for 10 minutes.

While crust is baking, combine all filling ingredients in a food processor until well incorporated.

When done, remove crust from oven and pour filling evenly over top.

Continue to bake for 15-20 minutes, or until filling is set, but still has a little jiggle.

Cool completely on wire rack. (You can also chill in the fridge if desired, to further set the filling).

168. Gorgeous Berry Smoothie

Ingredients:
½ cup frozen blueberries or 1 cup fresh blueberries
15 oz coconut milk
Stevia to taste
1 scoop of hemp protein
¼ teaspoon cinnamon (optional)

Instructions:
Place all ingredients into a blender.

Blend until mixed thoroughly.

Serve right away.

169. Tempting Coconut Berry Smoothie

Ingredients:
½ Cup Frozen Blackberries
½ Frozen Banana
1 Teaspoon Chia Seeds
¼ Inch Piece of Fresh Ginger
½ Cup Almond
Coconut Milk
1 scoop of HEMP protein
2 Tablespoons Toasted Coconut

Instructions:
Combine all the ingredients in a blender and process until smooth.

170. Volumptious Vanilla Hot Drink

Ingredients:
3 cups unsweetened almond milk (or 1 1/2 cup full fat coconut milk + 1 1/2 cups water)
Stevia to taste
1 scoop of hemp protein
1/2 Tbsp. ground cinnamon (or more to taste)
1/2 Tbsp. vanilla extract

Instructions:
Place the almond milk into a pitcher. Place ground cinnamon, hemp, anilla extract in a small saucepan over medium high heat. Heat until the pure liquid stevia is just melted and then pour the pure liquid stevia mixture into the pitcher.

Stir until the pure liquid stevia is well combined with the almond milk. Place the pitcher in the fridge and allow to chill for at least two hours. Stir well before serving.

171. Almond Butter Smoothies

Ingredients:
1 scoop of hemp protein
1 Tablespoon natural almond butter
1 cup of hemp milk
1 banana, preferably frozen for a creamier shake
few ice cubes

Instructions:
Blend all ingredients together and enjoy!

172. Choco Walnut Delight

Ingredients:
1 scoop Hemp Protein
30g dark sugar free chocolate broken up.
50g walnuts chopped/crushed (depending on desired texture)
250ml hemp milk or nut milk alternative
Handfull of ice cubes, the more you use the thicker it will be.

Instructions:
Blend everything together in a strong blender until thoroughly processed, and enjoy!

Makes 2, and can be stored in the fridge overnight.

173. Raspberry Hemp Smoothie

Ingredients:
1 cup hemp milk or milk alternative
1/2 cup raspberries (fresh or frozen)
2 tablespoons hemp protein powder
Stevia to taste
3 to 4 ice cubes

Instructions:
Add ingredients to a blender and blend until smooth.

174. Choco Banana Smoothie

Ingredients:
1 cup milk or milk alternative
2 peeled frozen bananas
4 ice cubes
2 tablespoons hulled hemp seed
2 tablespoons hemp protein powder
1 tablespoons organic cocoa powder
5-7 drops liquid stevia to sweeten
1/4 teaspoon cinnamon
1/4 teaspoon vanilla

Instructions:
Put all ingredients into blender. Blend until smooth.

175. Blueberry Almond Smoothie

Ingredients:
1 c almond milk
1 c frozen unsweetened blueberries
1 Tbsp cold-pressed organic flaxseed oil
2 tblsp hemp protein powder

Instructions:
Combine milk and blueberries in blender, and blend for 1 minute.

Transfer to glass, and stir in flaxseed oil.

176. Hazelnut Butter and Banana Smoothie

Ingredients:
½ c nut milk
½ c hemp milk
2 Tbsp creamy natural unsalted hazelnut butter
¼ very ripe banana
stevia drops to taste
4 ice cubes
2 tblsp hemp protein powder

Instructions:
Combine ingredients in a blender. Process until smooth.

Pour into a tall glass and serve.

177. Vanilla Blueberry Smoothie

Ingredients:
2 cups hemp milk
1 c fresh blueberries
Handful of ice OR 1 cup frozen blueberries
1 Tbsp flaxseed oil
2 tblsp hemp protein powder

Instructions:
Combine milk, and fresh blueberries plus ice (or frozen blueberries) in a blender.

Blend for 1 minute, transfer to a glass, and stir in flaxseed oil.

178. Chocolate Raspberry Smoothie

Ingredients:
1 cup almond milk
¼ c chocolate chips-sugar free
1 c fresh raspberries
2 tsp hemp protein powder
Handful of ice OR 1 cup frozen raspberries

Instructions:
COMBINE ingredients in a blender.

Blend for 1 minute, transfer to a glass, and eat with a spoon.

179. Peach Smoothie

Ingredients:
1 cup hemp milk
1 c frozen unsweetened peaches
2 tsp cold-pressed organic flaxseed oil (MUFA)
2 tsp hemp protein powder

Instructions:
PLACE milk and frozen, unsweetened peaches in blender and blend for 1 minute.

Transfer to glass, and stir in flaxseed oil.

180. Zesty Citrus Smoothie

Ingredients:
1 cup almond milk
half cup lemon juice
1 med orange peeled, cleaned, and sliced into sections
Handful of ice
1 Tbsp flaxseed oil
2 tsp hemp protein powder

Instructions:
COMBINE milk, lemon juice, orange, and ice in a blender.

Blend for 1 minute, transfer to a glass, and stir in flaxseed oil.

181. Apple Smoothie

Ingredients:
½ cup hemp milk
1 cup hemp milk
1 tsp apple pie spice
1 med apple peeled and chopped
2 Tbsp cashew butter
Handful of ice
2 tblsp hemp protein powder

Instructions:
COMBINE ingredients in a blender.

Blend for 1 minute, transfer to a glass, and eat with a spoon.

182. Pineapple Smoothie

Ingredients:
1 cup almond milk
4 oz fresh pineapple
Handful of ice
2 tblsp hemp protein powder
1 Tbsp cold-pressed organic flaxseed oil

Instructions:
PLACE milk, canned pineapple in blender, add of ice, and whip for 1 minute.

Transfer to glass and stir in flaxseed oil.

183. Strawberry Smoothie

Ingredients:
1 cup almond milk
1 c frozen, unsweetened strawberries
2 tblsp hemp protein powder
2 tsp cold-pressed organic flaxseed oil

Instructions:
COMBINE milk and strawberries in blender.

Blend, transfer to glass, and stir in flaxseed oil.

184. Pineapple Coconut Deluxe Smoothie

Ingredients:
1 C pineapple chunks
1 C coconut milk
1/2 C pineapple juice
1 ripe banana
1/2 – 3/4 C ice cubes
Pure liquid stevia to taste
1 tablespoon hemp protein powder

Instructions:

In a blender, combine the pineapple chunks, coconut milk, banana, ice and pure liquid stevia.

Puree until smooth.

Pour into 2 large glasses.

Garnish with a pineapple wedge if desired.

185. Divine Vanilla Smoothie

Ingredients:
1 cup coconut or almond milk
¼ cup almond butter
1 tsp vanilla paste, (or vanilla extract)
2 cups ice
Vanilla liquid, seeds or powder, to taste
Vanilla or plain hemp Protein Powder – 1 tablespoon

Instructions:
Add all ingredients except ice to blender. Puree well.

Add ice and blend until ice is all crushed and smoothie is well blended and smooth.

Pour into two glasses and serve immediately.

NOTES
Add more or less ice to make the smoothie thinner or thicker consistency. Great for a post workout smoothie!

186. Coco Orange Delish Smoothie

Ingredients:
1/2 cup fresh squeezed orange juice (I used 1 1/2 oranges)
1 tablespoon hemp protein powder
1/2 cup full fat coconut milk from the can (not the box!)
1 teaspoon vanilla
1/2 -1 cup crushed ice

Instructions:
Add all ingredients to a blender.

Blend until smooth and add ice as needed to get the consistency you like.

187. Baby Kale Pineapple Smoothie

Ingredients:
1 cup almond milk
1/2 cup frozen pineapple
1 cup Kale
1 tablespoon hemp protein powder

Instructions:
Place the almond milk, pineapple, and greens in the blender and blend until smooth.

188. Sumptuous Strawberry Coconut Smoothie

Ingredients:
1 cup coconut milk
1 frozen banana, sliced
2 cups frozen strawberries
1 teaspoon vanilla extract
1 tablespoon hemp protein powder

Instructions:
Add all ingredients to blender and blend until smooth.

189. Blueberry Bonanza Smoothies

Ingredients:
1/4 cup canned coconut or almond milk
1/2 cup water
1 medium banana, sliced
1 cup frozen blueberries
1 tablespoon raw almonds

Instructions:
Add coconut milk, water, banana, blueberries and almonds to blender container.

Cover and blend until smooth. Pour into 2 glasses.

190. Divine Peach Coconut Smoothie

Ingredients:
1 cup full fat coconut milk, chilled
1 cup ice
2 large fresh peaches, peeled and cut into chunks
Fresh lemon zest, to taste
1 tablespoon hemp protein powder

Instructions:
Add coconut milk, ice and peaches blender. Using a zester, add a few gratings of fresh lemon zest.

Blend on high speed until smooth.

191. Tantalizing Key Lime Pie Smoothie

Ingredients:
1 cup coconut milk
1 cup ice
1/2 avocado
zest and juice of 2 limes
Pure liquid stevia to taste
1 tablespoon hemp protein powder

Instructions:
Add all ingredients to Vitamix or blender and blend until smooth.

192. High Protein and Nutritional Delish Smoothie

Ingredients:
1 cup almond milk
1/2 Avocado
4 Strawberries
1/2 Bananas (Very ripe)
1/2 cup Raw Kale or spinach
1/4 cup Carrot Juice) water can be used
1 cup Coconut Yogurt..or almond milk)
1 tablespoon hemp protein powder

Instructions:
Add everything to your blender, and blend to your preferred consistency

More water or ice can be added to help with your preferred texture/thickness.

193. Pineapple Protein Smoothie

Ingredients:
1 cup (135g) pineapple chunks
1 cup (200g) coconut milk (fresh or tinned)
½ med (65g) banana
¼ cup (65g) ice cubes
¼ tsp vanilla bean powder
pinch low sodium salt
1 tablespoon hemp protein powder

Instructions:
Peel pineapple and chop into small chunks.

Put everything into a high speed blender and blend until smooth.

194. Raspberry Coconut Smoothie

Ingredients:
½ - 1 cup coconut milk (depending on how thick you like it)
1 medium banana, peeled sliced and frozen
2 teaspoons coconut extract (optional)
1 cup frozen raspberries
1 tablespoon hemp protein powder

optional: shredded coconut flakes, and stevia to taste

Instructions:
Add coconut milk, frozen banana slices and coconut extract to your blender.

Pulse 1-2 minutes until smooth.

Add frozen raspberries and continue to pulse until smooth.

Pour into your serving glass, top with a couple of raspberries and a little shredded coconut, and enjoy!

195. Ginger Carrot Protein Smoothie

Ingredients:
3/4 cup carrot juice
1 tablespoon hemp protein powder
1 tablespoon hulled hemp seeds
1/2 apple
3 to 4 ice cubes
1/2 inch piece fresh ginger

Instructions:
Add to a blender and blend until smooth.

196. Delish Banana Nut Muffins

Ingredients:
4 bananas, mashed with a fork (the more ripe, the better)
4 eggs
1/2 cup almond butter
2 tbsp coconut oil, melted
1 tsp vanilla
1/2 cup coconut flour
2 tsp cinnamon
1/2 tsp nutmeg
1 tsp baking powder
1 tsp baking soda
1/4 tsp low sodium salt

Instructions:
Preheat oven to 350 degrees F. Line a muffin tin with cups. In a large bowl, add bananas, eggs, almond butter, coconut oil, and vanilla. Using a hand blender, blend to combine.

Add in the coconut flour, cinnamon, nutmeg, baking powder, baking soda, and low sodium salt. Blend into the wet mixture, scraping down the sides with a spatula. Distribute the batter evenly into the lined muffin tins, filling each about two-thirds of the way full.

Bake for 20-25 minutes, until a toothpick comes out clean. Serve warm or store in the refrigerator in a resealable bag.

197. Delightful Cinnamon Apple Muffins

Ingredients:
1 cup unsweetened applesauce
4 eggs
1/4 cup coconut oil, melted
1 tsp vanilla
Stevia to taste
1/2 cup coconut flour
2 tsp cinnamon
1 tsp baking powder
1 tsp baking soda
1/4 tsp low sodium salt

Instructions:

Preheat oven to 350 degrees F. Line a muffin tin with liners. In a large bowl, add applesauce, eggs, coconut oil, stevia, and vanilla. Stir to combine.

Stir in the coconut flour, cinnamon, baking powder, baking soda, and low sodium salt. Distribute the batter evenly into the lined muffin tins, filling each about two-thirds of the way full.

Bake for 15-20 minutes, until a toothpick inserted into the center comes out clean. Serve warm or store in the refrigerator in a resealable bag.

198. Healthy Breakfast Bonanza Muffins

Ingredients:
8 eggs
1 cup diced broccoli
1 cup diced onion
1 cup diced mushrooms
low sodium salt and pepper, to taste
This recipe makes 8 muffins.

Instructions:
Preheat oven to 350 degrees F.

Dice all vegetables. You can add more or less of any of them, but keep the overall portion of vegetables the same for best results.

In a large mixing bowl, whisk together eggs, vegetables, low sodium salt, and pepper.

Pour mixture into a greased muffin pan, the mixture should evenly fill 8 muffin cups.

Bake 18-20 minutes, or until a toothpick inserted in the middle comes out clean.

Serve and enjoy! Leftovers can be saved in the refrigerator throughout the week.

199. Perfect Pumpkin Seeds

Ingredients:
1 cup of pumpkin (only seeds)
2 teaspoons of olive oil
1 tablespoon of chili powder (you may adjust it as per the taste you like)
1 teaspoon low sodium salt

Instructions:
Heat the pan (medium high heat) and place the pumpkin seeds.

After 3 to 5 minutes, you will hear the seeds making a crackling noise (some will even pop). You need to stir frequently.

Remove the pan and mix the seeds in olive oil, then low sodium salt and chili powder. Let it cool and then serve.

200. Gorgeous Spicy Nuts

Ingredients:
2/3 cup of each (almonds, pecans and walnuts)
1 teaspoon of chili powder
½ teaspoon of cumin
½ teaspoon of black
pepper (ground)
½ teaspoon low sodium salt
1 tables

Instructions:
Heat the pan on medium heat and place the nuts and toast them until lightly browned.

Prepare the spice mixture, while the nuts are toasting.

Mix cumin, chili, low sodium salt and black pepper in a bowl and add the nuts (after coating it with olive oil).

201. Krunchy Yummy Kale Chips

Ingredients:
1 bunch of kale, washed and dried
2 tbsp olive oil
low sodium salt to taste

Instructions:
Preheat oven to 300 degrees. Remove the center stems and either tear or cut up the leaves.

Toss the kale and olive oil together in a large bowl; sprinkle with low sodium salt. Spread on a baking sheet

Bake at 300 degrees for 15 minutes or until crisp.

202. Delicious Cinnamon Apple Chips

Ingredients:
1-2 apples
1 tsp cinnamon

Instructions:
Preheat oven to 200 degrees.

Using a sharp knife or mandolin, slice apples thinly. Discard seeds. Prepare a baking sheet with parchment paper and arrange apple slices on it without overlapping. Sprinkle cinnamon over apples.

Bake for approximately 1 hour, then flip. Continue baking for 1-2 hours, flipping occasionally, until the apple slices are no longer moist. Store in airtight container.

203. Gummy Citrus Snack

Ingredients:
3/4 cup lemon juice, freshly squeezed* and ¼ cup apple juice freshly squeezed
4 Tbsp. good quality vegetarian gelatin
liquid stevia to taste
1/4 tsp. ginger (freshly grated or ground)
1/4 tsp. turmeric (freshly grated or ground)

Instructions:
In a small saucepan, whisk together citrus juice, and gelatin until there are no lumps. Heat the liquid over low heat until liquid is warmed and gelatin is completely dissolved.

Remove from heat and stir in liquid stevia, ginger and turmeric with a spoon.

Pour into a casserole dish*.

Refrigerate until liquid is set (at least 30 minutes).

Serve cold or at room temperature.

204. Skinny Veggie Dip

Ingredients:
1 tblsp olive oil
1 tsp lemon juice
1 Tbs fresh minced parsley
1 Tbs french minced chives or scallion greens
1 tsp dried dill
1/8 tsp garlic powder
Pinch paprika
low sodium salt and pepper to taste

Instructions:
Combine in triple portions in blender and store to use any time.

205. Divine Butternut Chips

Ingredients:
1 medium butternut squash (400g / 14.1 oz)
2 tbsp extra virgin coconut oil
1 tsp gingerbread spice mix (~ ½ tsp cinnamon, pinch nutmeg, ginger, cloves and allspice)
pinch low sodium salt (or more in case you don't use stevia and prefer the chips salty)
optional: 3-6 drops liquid Stevia extract

Instructions:
Preheat the oven to 125 C / 250 F. Peel the butternut squash and slice thinly on a mandolin. If you are using a knife, make sure the slices are no more than 1/8 inch (1/4 cm) thin. Place in a bowl.

In a small bowl, mix melted coconut oil, gingerbread spice mix and stevia.

Pour the oil mixture over the butternut squash and mix well to allow it everywhere.

Arrange the slices close to each other on a baking tray lined with parchment paper or a rack or an oven chip tray (you will need at least 2 of them).

Place in the oven and cook for about 1.5 hour or until crispy (the exact time depends on how thick the chips are).

206. Outstanding Orange Skinny Snack

Ingredients:
1 T. vanilla extract
½ t. natural orange flavor
Pinch low sodium salt
1 ½ t. liquid stevia to taste
8 T. vegetarian gelatin
1 can coconut milk
1 ½ C. water

Instructions:
Heat water and coconut milk over low heat until simmering.

Continue on low heat, slowly adding in each tablespoon of gelatin, whisking the entire time.

Add remaining ingredients and whisk until any clumps of gelatin are gone.

Pour into molds, and pour remaining liquid into 8X8 glass pan.

Put in fridge until solid. …should pop out easily once hardened.

207. Spicy Pumpkin Seed Bonanza

Ingredients:
1 1/2 cups pumpkin seeds,
3 jalapeño peppers, sliced
3 tablespoons olive oil
low sodium salt and paprika, to taste

Instructions:
Preheat the oven to 350°F

Spread pumpkin seeds out on a rimmed baking sheet.

Add olive oil and low sodium salt and stir pumpkin seeds with your hands to combine.

Lay slices of jalapeño peppers on top of seeds.

Sprinkle paprika over the top of everything, generously.

Bake for 10 minutes.

Use a spatula to move the seeds and peppers around. Bake for another 5 minutes.

Move mixture around some more and bake for a final 5 minutes.

Remove tray from oven and let everything rest for 15-30 minutes to let the jalapeño-ness soak into the seeds.

Store in an airtight container...if you don't finish them all in one sitting.

208. Delectable Chocolate-Frosted Doughnuts

Ingredients:
For the doughnuts:
1 tbsp water, separated into 1/2 tablespoons
3 eggs
1 tsp vanilla
1/4 cup coconut flour
1/4 cup coconut oil, melted
1 tbsp cinnamon
1/4 tsp baking soda
low sodium salt to taste

For the frosting:
1/2 cup sugar free dairy free Chocolate Chips
1 tbsp coconut oil

Instructions:

Turn on donut hole maker (You could also make these into regular donuts and cook at 350 for about 15 or so minutes).

Combine eggs, and vanilla in a food processor until well combined.

Add in the rest of the ingredients and continue to process until all ingredients are incorporated.

Add appropriate amount of batter to donut hole maker and use as instructed (Mine took about 3 or so minutes for each batch, but this will vary for different types).

While your donuts are baking, prepare the frosting by combing chocolate chips and coconut oil over LOW heat until melted.

Once donuts are completely cooled, dip each in frosting with a toothpick or skewer and completely cover, tapping off excess frosting. (I used a longer skewer stick and placed them standing up in a cup to harden, but if you aren't concerned with appearance, you can dip them with a fork or spoon, even, and just place them on a plate).

Place donuts in refrigerator to completely harden (about 1 hour).

209. Eggplant Divine

Ingredients:
1 large eggplant (about 1 pound)
1/2 cup olive oil
4 tablespoons balsamic vinegar
2 tablespoons pure liquid stevia
1/2 teaspoon paprika
low sodium salt

Instructions:
Wash eggplant and slice into thin strips. For ease in snacking you can cut long strips in half crosswise. Leave full-length for a more bacon-like appearance.

In a large bowl whisk together oil, vinegar, stevia, and paprika. Place strips in the mixture a few at a time, turning to make sure each is completely coated. If you run short of marinade, add a little more oil and stir it in with your hands.

Marinate 2 hours. Then, place strips on baking sheets

To dry in the oven: Line one or two rimmed baking sheets with parchment paper. Lay strips on sheets, close together but not overlapping. Sprinkle on a little low sodium salt (you don't need much).

Place in oven on lowest setting for 10 to 12 hours (ovens' lowest setting varies, thus drying time will vary) or until dry and fairly crisp, turning strips partway through. Check occasionally, and if any oil pools on the sheets, blot with a paper towel.

210. Choco Apple Nachos

Ingredients:
apples
fresh lemon juice
almond butter
chocolate chips
unsweetened shredded coconut
sliced almonds

Instructions:
Slice apples and toss with the lemon juice in a large bowl.

Arrange the apples in a plate and drizzle with almond butter. You can use a pastry/piping bag or a ziplock bag to drizzle the almond butter.

Sprinkle with shredded coconut, chocolate chips and sliced almonds.

211. Skinny Delicious Snack Bars

Ingredients:
1/2 cup almond butter
1 cup (250 grams) cooled roast pumpkin or pumpkin puree
3 cups desiccated coconut (finely shredded dried coconut)
1 (150 grams) ripe banana
1 teaspoon cinnamon
1 teaspoon vanilla
pinch of low sodium salt

Instructions:
Preheat your oven to 175 Degrees Celsius or 350 Degrees Fahrenheit.

Grease and line a 20cm x 20cm square cake tin with baking paper hanging over the sides for easy removal.

Place all ingredients into your blender or food processor in the order listed, blend to combine.

Press the mixture into the tin and cook for 30 minutes or until golden on top and an inserted skewer comes out cleanly.

Remove from the oven, leave in the tin for five minutes then carefully move the slice onto a cooling rack. Once it has cooled chop into bars. Enjoy!

212. Pumpkin Vanilla Delight

Ingredients:
115g (1/2 cup) pumpkin seeds
1 tsp vanilla extract
2 tsp liquid stevia
Water (boiled)

Instructions:
Preheat oven to 150c.

In a medium bowl, combine the liquid stevia, and vanilla. Stir together to create a thick paste then add a small drop of boiled water to thin it out and create a runny syrup.

Pour in the pumpkin seeds and stir them around in the mixture to evenly coat them.

Dollop a generous tsp full of the pumpkin seeds onto a baking sheet, repeat until it's all used up and cook for 15-20 minutes until most of the seeds have browned (but don't let them burn!)

Take out of the oven and leave to cool for a few minutes. Once they've cooled a little (but are still warm) you can press the clusters together to make sure they don't fall apart. They will dry quickly.

Once they're cooled and dried, they're ready to eat! Enjoy on their own or served on top of your cereal.

213. Skinny Quicky Crackers

Ingredients:
1 heaped cup of almond meal
1 egg
2 teaspoons olive oil
Pinch of low sodium salt

Instructions:
Preheat your oven to 180 degrees Celsius or 350 degrees Fahrenheit.

Place your ingredients into your blender or food processor in the order listed above, quickly combine at medium speed – you don't want the mixture to become sticky or turn to almond butter, although do not worry if this happens, it will still work.

Roll the mixture into a ball and place between two sheets of baking paper, roll out to your desired thickness.

Remove the top layer of baking paper and place on an oven tray. Bake for 20 minutes or until nicely golden. Remove from the oven and allow to cool prior to cutting into crackers. Enjoy.

214. Delectable Parsnip Chips

Ingredients:

500g (1.1 pounds) Parsnips
1/4 Cup Coconut Oil, Melted
3 Tablespoons liquid stevia

Instructions:

Preheat the oven to 200°C (392°F) and get out an oven proof dish.

Peel the parsnips and cut them into chip sized pieces and place into the oven proof dish.

Pour over the coconut oil and distribute evenly.

Drizzle over the liquid stevia and stir to combine well.

Place in the oven and cook for 15 minutes.

Remove from the oven and toss the parsnips over to allow the other side to brown.

Place back in the oven and cook for a further 10 to 15 minutes or until golden.

215. Spicy Crunchy Skinny Snack

Ingredients:
3/4 cup almond flour
1/4 cup coconut flour
1/4 cup flax seeds
1/4 cup of olive oil
1/2 tsp low sodium salt
1 1/2 tsp chilli
1/2 tsp cumin
1/2 tsp paprika powder
1 egg
1/2 tsp garlic powder

Instructions:
Melt the butter and basically mix up all the ingredients together, and knead it into a ball.

Take 2 sheets of baking paper, lay the ball on one, the other sheet on top and then flatten it out with a roller.

Cut triangles with a knife. Heat the oven to about 180C (350F) and bake for about 10 mins. Keep an eye on them so they don't burn.

216. Raw Hemp Kale Bars

Ingredients:
1/2 cup pistachios
1/2 cup pumpkin seeds
3/4 cup shredded coconut
1/4 cup orange juice
1/4 cup hemp seeds
1/4 cup coconut oil, melted
¼ cup dried kale crunched
3/4 cup dates, chopped

Instructions:

In a food processor, process the pistachios, pumpkin seeds, shredded coconut and dates until the mixture is crumbly but beginning to come together.

Remove to a medium mixing bowl and stir in orange juice, coconut oil, hemp seeds and kale.

Press into an 8-inch square cake pan or glass dish.

Chill in the refrigerator for at least an hour, then slice and serve.

217. Skinny Trail Mix

Ingredients:
1 cup flaked unsweetened coconut
1/2 cup raw almonds
1/2 cup raw pecans or walnuts
1/2 cup raw pumpkin seeds
1/2 cup raw sunflower seeds
1/2 cup dairy free sugar free Chocolate Chips

Instructions:
Combine all ingredients in a large mixing bowl and toss to combine.

Divide the trail mix between 9 sandwich baggies (about 1/2 cup of mix per bag) for a handy snack.

218. Anti-Aging Fruit Delights

Ingredients:
1 1/4 – 1/2 cups of pureed strawberries and raspberries
*If you prefer a less concentrated version, use 1 1/4 c fruit puree, and 1/4 c water!
4 – 5 tbsp vegetarian **gelatin**

Instructions:

Pureé the strawberries and raspberries.

In a small pan or pot on medium heat, whisk the gelatin into the fruit pureé until the gelatin is fully dissolved.

Pour the mixture into a glass pan. The smaller the size, the thicker the fruit snacks.

Chill the mixture for about 30 – 45 minutes in the fridge.

Cut into pieces and enjoy! Store in the fridge.

219. Paleo Rosemary Sweet Potato Crunches

Ingredients:
2 large sweet potatoes, peeled
1 Tbls coconut oil, melted
1 tsp low sodium salt
2 tsp dried rosemary

Instructions:
Heat oven to 375 degrees.

Slice sweet potatoes using a mandolin set to 1/8th inch.

Grind low sodium salt and rosemary with a mortar and pestle.

Toss sweet potatoes in a bowl with coconut oil and low sodium salt -seasoning mixture.

Place on a non-stick baking sheet (or a regular pan greased with coconut oil) and place into the oven.

After 10 minutes, take the pan out and flip the chips.

Place chips back in for another 10 minutes.

Pull the pan out and place any chips that are starting to brown on a cooling rack.

Place the chips back in for 3-5 minutes. Every oven is different so keep a close eye on the chips so they don't burn.

Place remaining chips on the cooling rack.

220. Apple Peach Skinny Bars

Ingredients:
6 Eggs
liquid stevia to taste
1 tbs (15 mL) Coconut Oil
1/2 tsp (2.5 mL) Vanilla Extract
1/3 cup (40 g) Coconut Flour
1/4 tsp (1.25 mL) Baking Soda, optional
1/4 tsp (1.25 mL) low sodium salt
2 tbs (30 mL) Applesauce
1/2 Peach, diced
1/2 Apple, diced
1/8 tsp (1 mL) Nutmeg
1/8 tsp (1 mL) Ginger
1/4 tsp (1.25 mL) Cinnamon

Instructions:
Preheat your oven to 325° F (163° C).
Grease an 8x8 inch pan (20x20 cm square) and line it with parchment paper.
Puree the eggs, liquid stevia, coconut oil, applesauce, and vanilla in a food processor or blender.
Add the coconut flour, baking soda, low sodium salt, and spices and blend until smooth.
Fold in the apple and peach
Pour the batter into the prepared pan and bake for 35-40 min or until a toothpick inserted into the center comes out clean.

221. Spicy Fried Almonds

Ingredients:
2 cups raw almonds, blanched*-boil for 3 minutes
2 tablespoons fresh rosemary, minced
2 teaspoons low sodium salt (or to taste, depending on how salty you like nuts)
coconut oil, or olive oil**

Instructions:
Heat a large pan over medium heat.

Add enough oil to generously coat the bottom of your pan (approx. 3-4 tablespoons), and allow to heat up.

Add the almonds to the pan. Stir frequently so that the almonds don't burn. The almonds will be ready when they're golden brown (approx. 5-7 minutes).

Turn down the heat to low and add the rosemary and low sodium salt. Stir well, and cook just until the rosemary becomes fragrant (approx. 2 minutes).

Remove the almonds from the pan and place on paper towel to drain any remaining oil.

Enjoy warm or once cooled.

222. Zucchini Avocado Hummus

Ingredients:
1 zucchini courgette, peeled and diced small
1/4 avocado (a generous tbsp's worth)
1 clove garlic
2 tsps lemon juice
1 tsp cumin
3 tsps tahini
1 tsp extra virgin olive oil

Instructions:
Stick all the ingredients into a blender and pulse until smooth.

Dust with paprika to serve and keep in the fridge for 4- 5 days.

223. Skinny Power Snack

Ingredients:
1/2 Avocado
1/2 tsp Paprika
1/2 tsp low sodium salt
1/2 tsp Garlic Powder

Instructions:
Sprinkle with all the seasonings and enjoy.

224. Skinny Salsa

Add any of the crunchy chip recipes mentioned in this book

Ingredients:
1 red onion, peeled and quartered
1/4 cup roasted hot New Mexico green chiles
6 large garlic cloves, still in skin
1/2 cup cilantro, chopped
1 qt cherry tomatoes
low sodium salt, to taste

Instructions:

Let the garlic roast for 5-7 minutes in a 200 degree oven. When the skins begin to darken, turn them over and continue to cook another 3 minutes.

Remove the garlic from the grill.

Now, place the tomatoes and onion in the grill Roast the veggies until nicely charred.

While the veggies are roasting, peel the garlic. Place the garlic in a food processor. When the veggies are finished roasting on the grill, add the tomatoes to the food processor along with the roasted New Mexico chiles and low sodium salt. Pulse to form a chunky puree. Pour into a mixing bowl.

Now, hand dice the onions and add the cilantro. Stir to incorporate and adjust seasoning, as necessary.

Pour into a serving vessel surrounded by your choice of skinny chips. Serve & enjoy.

225. Divine Turkey Stuffed Tomatoes

Ingredients:
2 lbs small tomatoes (bigger than cherry tomatoes, but small enough that you can eat them in two bites)
1 lb cooked turkey meat, chopped or shredded
2-3 stalks celery, finely chopped
3 Tbs minced red onion
1 carrot, peeled and shredded
low sodium salt and pepper to taste

Instructions:
Add the all ingredients other than the tomatoes and mix thoroughly. Taste and season with low sodium salt and pepper.

Cut a thin slice off the stem end of each tomato. Scoop out the insides (you can use your fingers but I used one of these scoops). Fill the tomatoes with turkey mix

Combine all ingredients. Refrigerate until serving.

226. Curried Nutty Delish

Ingredients:
2 Tablespoons organic curry powder
1 Tablespoon low sodium salt
liquid stevia to taste
2 Tablespoons water
1 Teaspoon olive oil
3 cups raw cashews, whole or pieces

Instructions:
Preheat the oven to 250F and line a baking sheet with parchment paper.

Mix together the first five ingredients and toss with the cashews.

Spread the nuts in an even layer and roast for 35-40 minutes.

Transfer to an airtight container. I made a bigger batch and put most of it in the freezer.

227. Skinny Chips

Ingredients:
1 (sweet potato) peeled and diced small
3 Small Parsnips peeled and diced small
4 lg cloves of garlic
1/2 Red Capsicum diced small
1 cup Flax meal
3 tbsp Chai seeds
1 tbsp Cumin seeds
1 tsp Smoked Paprika
1tsp low sodium salt
2 tbsp Olive Oil

Instructions:
Pre-heat oven 170c.

Place your raw diced sweet potato, parsnips, red capsicum, garlic and olive oil in your food processor and blend until into a fine mash.

Now that your raw vegetables are a mash add the rest of your ingredients. Blend in your food processor until well combined.

I then cut my dough into chip shapes with a knife on my oven tray. The key is to cut down rather that slice through.

I placed my ready cut "chips" in the oven. I pulled them out after 7 minutes and flipped them over.

After that every 3-4 minutes I turned them. I continued this over 20 minutes. (ovens will vary) I then turned my oven down to its lowest temp to dry them out further. This took a further 10 minutes. Remember each oven is different just ensure you have plenty of time during the cooking period to check and turn as needed. My oven isn't fan bake its old. So yours may crisp up faster!

228. Zesty Zucchini Pesto Roll-ups

Ingredients:
2 zucchinis
1 container of cherry tomatoes
1/2 c. pesto

For the Pesto:
1 c. fresh basil leaves
2 Tbsp. minced garlic
3/4 c. raw cashews
2 Tbsp. freshly squeezed lemon juice
1/3 c. olive oil
1 tsp. low sodium salt

Instructions:
Start off by making the pesto – mainly because it becomes more flavorful the longer it sits. Combine cashews, olive oil, basil, garlic, lemon juice, nutritional yeast, low sodium salt, and pepper in a food processor. Pulse until the consistency is mostly smooth. Cover and refrigerate.

Chop the ends off each zucchini. Then, using a mandolin or vegetable peeler, start peeling long strips from the zucchini. Repeat until you've peeled enough strips for the amount of rolls you want to make.

Have the cherry tomatoes ready in a bowl and a stockpile of toothpicks. On a flat surface, lay out a slice of zucchini, portion a spoonful on the strip and smooth it out evenly. Cover 1/2-3/4 of the strip, otherwise it will be hard to roll and the pesto will ooze out everywhere. Place a cherry tomato near one end of the zucchini and start to roll the strip around the tomato. When you get to the end, spear the roll with a toothpick and set it aside.

229. Butternut Squash-raw Veggie Dip

Ingredients:
1 cup cooked and peeled squash
½ cup COCONUT cream
½ teaspoon low sodium salt
1 teaspoon olive oil
1 ½ teaspoons finely chopped shallot
2 teaspoons fresh thyme
¼ teaspoon ground cinnamon
1 teaspoon chili powder

Instructions:
Place squash in a medium bowl and smash with a fork. Add remaining ingredients, mixing until thoroughly combined.

Serve dip with carrot sticks, veggies, or SKINNY CHIPS.

230. Skinny Power Balls

Ingredients:
1 medium size cooked sweet potato
2 cups almond meal
1 tsp vanilla powder
3 tsp baking powder
3 egg yolks
4 Tbsp melted Coconut Oil
liquid stevia to taste
3 Tbsp coconut flour (I used Coconut Secret brand)
1 cup of unsweetened shredded coconut and coconut flakes

Instructions:

Peel and mash cooked sweet potato until no more chunks left.

Mix in almond meal, vanilla powder, baking powder until everything incorporates.

Mix in the wet ingredients (egg yolks, melted coconut oil and liquid stevia), stir until everything combines.

Add 3 Tbsp coconut flour. Notice the mixture will be less wet but not too dry. Do not try to put too much coconut flour as it absorbs a lot of moisture and the balls would be too dry and flaky.

Line a baking sheet with a parchment paper. Pre-heat the oven for 350°F

Shape the balls into ping-pong ball size and roll each of them in the bowl of unsweetened shredded coconut and coconut flakes.

Bake the balls in 350°F for about 25 minutes or until the edges turned golden brown or they are dried out already. Remove from heat and let them cool down. The balls are soft when they're still warm but as they cooled down, they should be more firm. After they cooled down, put them in a fridge so they'll be more firm.

231. Chocolate Goji Skinny Bars

Ingredients:
1 cup raw cashews
1/2 cup cocoa powder
1/2 cup dried goji berries
1/2 cup hemp seeds
1 cup shredded coconut
2-3 tbsp coconut oil
liquid stevia to taste

Instructions:
Process cashews in a food processor until it turns into a paste. Roasted cashews don't work as well because they are less sticky.

Transfer paste into a large mixing bowl. Put coconut oil and liquid stevia into another smaller bowl and warm in the oven until it is fully melted.

While this is heating up, add the dried coconut, cocoa powder, and goji berries to the mixing bowl

Transfer melted coconut oil and liquid stevia into mixing bowl.

Everything should now be in the mixing bowl except for the hemp seeds. Mix everything in the bowl with a fork or your hands until thoroughly combined.

This should make a fairly mold-able dough. Spread the hemp seeds onto a plate. Begin to form your dough into small bite-sized balls and then roll them in the hemp seeds until they are thoroughly coated.

Pop in the fridge for at least 2 hours to harden them up a bit.

232. Delish Cashew Butter Treats

Ingredients:
1 Cup Cashews
Half cup coconut flour
0.5 Cup Cashew Butter

Instructions:
Add the cashews and cashew butter and process until the mixture forms a dough ball.

Add coconut flour to harden the mixture. You may need to scrape down the sides and help the mixture along to form a dough ball.

Once a dough ball has formed, move the dough to a plate to ensure there are no accidents with the food processor blade.

Form the mixture into 16 equal sized balls, refrigerate for at least an hour to harden and enjoy!

233. Roasted Tasty Tomato Soup

Ingredients:
1 lb fresh tomatoes
1 red onion, medium
1 small head garlic, pealed
1 tbsp olive oil
1 tsp low sodium salt
1/2 tsp fresh cracked black pepper
1 tsp oregano
3/4 cup low sodium chicken broth, homemade preferably
15 oz tomato sauce, canned - sugar and salt free
chives to top

Instructions:
Preheat oven to 375 degrees F.

Cube tomatoes and onion. Place on baking sheet. Drizzle with olive oil and sprinkle with seasonings. Slice butter into small pieces on top of vegetables. Roast for 30 minutes, stirring halfway after 15 minutes.

Allow roasted vegetables to cool for 10 minutes. Purée vegetables, broth and tomato sauce in blender until smooth, scraping down the sides several times while blending.

Heat tomato soup in a sauce pan allowing the soup to slowly simmer for a few minutes to blend the flavors together. Serve hot topped with chives.

234. Thai Coconut Turkey Soup

Ingredients:
A small splash of oil
1 onion, sliced thin
A big handful of shiitake mushrooms, cut in half
3 cloves of garlic, finely minced
1 inch piece of ginger, julienned
A handful of cherry tomatoes
4 cups turkey stock 1 cup shredded cooked turkey (or chicken) meat
½ cup canned coconut milk
low sodium salt to taste
A small handful of cilantro

Instructions:
Stir fry onion, garlic, ginger and the add mushrooms and tomatoes.

Add turkey meat and fry for a few minutes till slightly browned.

Add stock and simmer for 20 minutes.

Serve warm and sprinkle chives on top.

235. Cheeky Chicken Soup

Ingredients:
2 large organic chicken breasts, skin removed and cut into ½ inch strips
1 28oz can of diced tomatoes
32 ounces low sodium organic chicken broth
1 sweet onion, diced
2 cups of shredded carrots
2 cups chopped celery
1 bunch of cilantro chopped fine
4 cloves of garlic, minced - I always use one of these
2 Tbs tomato paste
1 tsp chili powder
1 tsp cumin
low sodium salt & fresh cracked pepper to taste
olive oil
1-2 cups water

Instructions:
In a crockpot place a dash of olive oil and about ¼ cup chicken broth. Add onions, garlic, jalapeno, low sodium salt and pepper and cook until soft, adding more broth as needed.

Then add all of your remaining ingredients and enough water to fill to the top of your pot. Cover and let cook on low for about 2 hrs, adjusting low sodium salt & pepper as needed.

Once the chicken is fully cooked, you should be able to shred it very easily. I simply used the back of a wooden spoon and pressed the cooked chicken against the side of the pot.

Top with avocado slices and fresh cilantro. Enjoy!

236. Triple Squash Delight Soup

Ingredients:
1 butternut squash
1 gold acorn squash
1 white acorn squash
1-2 cups vegetable stock (depending on squash size, and how thick you want the soup)
2 cups diced turkey breast
1/4 cup light coconut milk
1 tbsp. olive oil
low sodium salt for seasoning

Instructions:
Preheat the oven to 400 degrees.

Halve each squash, scoop out the seeds (and saving them for toasting), and then slice into 1-1 1/2 inch thick crescents.

Spread the squash on an aluminum foil-lined baking sheet and coat lightly with the olive oil. Season with low sodium salt. Roast for about 30 minutes, or until golden brown (turning once mid-way through baking).

When the squash has cooled from the oven slightly, spoon off the meat from the skin.

In a medium to large pot, bring the turkey meat, the meat of all the squash and 1 1/2 cups of vegetable stock to a boil. Turn the heat to low and stir in the coconut milk.

Remove from heat to puree the soup. You can use an immersion blender, or transfer everything to a traditional blender.

Blend until smooth, adding any additional stock to achieve the consistency you like.

237. Ginger Carrot Delight Soup

Ingredients:
3 tbsp unsalted butter or coconut oil
1 1/2 pounds carrots (6-7 large carrots), sliced
2 cups chopped white or yellow onion
1 cup diced turkey breast
low sodium salt
2 teaspoons minced ginger
2 cups low sodium chicken stock
2 cups water
3 large strips of zest from an orange

Instructions:
Heat up the butter or coconut oil in a large soup pot.

Add the chopped carrots, turkey breast and onion to the pot and cook over medium heat for 5-10 minutes. Don't allow the carrots or onion to brown.

Add in the remaining ingredients (ginger, orange zest, water, and stock). The orange zest will be pulled out prior to puréeing so make sure they are in large, easy to identify strips rather than small pieces.

Bring to a boil then simmer for 10 minutes.

Remove orange zest strips.

Purée the mixture with an immersion blender. Or divide into 3-4 batches and blend in a regular blender.

I garnished my soup with a touch of olive oil and some freshly ground low sodium salt and pepper.

238. Wonderful Watercress Soup

Ingredients:
1 quart low sodium chicken stock
1 medium leek
1 bunch water cress
1 large onion
1/2 celeriac root skinned and chopped
2 cups diced chicken breast – organic
low sodium salt and pepper to taste

Instructions:

Gently heat the chicken stock in the pot.

In the fry pan sauté the onion, leek and celeriac until soft.

Place the onion, leek, chicken and celeriac in the pot of stock reserving 1/3 aside.

Season with low sodium salt and pepper.

Add the bunch of watercress and simmer a few minutes until it is wilted.

With the immersion blender blend the soup.

Add the chopped vegetables that you reserved, back into the pot.

239. Curried Butternut Soup

Ingredients:
2 medium butternut squash, cut in half lengthwise, seeds removed
(save for garnish)
1 cup diced chicken breast – organic
1 medium yellow onion, chopped
1 inch piece fresh ginger, peeled and diced or grated
1 tablespoon curry powder
1 can coconut milk (find BPA-free coconut milk)
1 1/2 C chicken broth
Coconut Oil
low sodium salt and pepper

Instructions:
Preheat oven to 425 degrees.

Melt a tablespoon of coconut oil in a roasting pan.

Place squash, cut side down in roasting pan.

Roast 45 minutes to an hour, or until fork tender.

Add ginger and curry powder and saute 2 more minutes.

Scoop flesh out of roasted squash and add to apple mixture. Stir to incorporate flavors.

Add coconut milk, chicken and chicken broth. Stir to incorporate ingredients and bring to a boil.

Simmer mixture, uncovered for 20 minutes.

Using either a high power mixer or an immersion blender, blend soup until it's smooth.

240. Celery Cashew Cream Soup

Ingredients:
300 grams celery, washed and chopped
1 small onion, chopped
1.5 tbsp olive oil
500 mls vegetable stock
40 grams cashew nuts
low sodium salt and pepper to taste

Instructions:
Heat the olive oil in a large saucepan then add the celery and onion, stir to coat with oil. Turn the heat low and put the lid on leaving the vegetables to sweat for 5 minutes.

Add the garlic, give a quick stir then add the vegetable stock and simmer for 10 minutes.

Add the cashew nuts to the saucepan and simmer for another 5 minutes or until the celery is cooked through.

Tip the soup mix into a blender and purée until smooth.

Season with the low sodium salt and pepper and serve.

241. Mighty Andalusian Gazpacho

Ingredients:
3 pounds very ripe tomatoes, cored and cut into chunks
½ pound cucumber, peeled, seeded, and cut chunks
⅓ pound red onion, peeled and cut into chunks
⅓ pound green or red bell pepper, cored, seeded, and cut into chunks
2 cloves garlic, peeled and smashed
1½ teaspoons low sodium salt, plus more to taste
1 cup extra-virgin olive oil, plus more for serving
2 tablespoons sherry vinegar, plus more for serving
2 tablespoons finely minced chives
Freshly ground black pepper

Instructions:
Put all veggies in a large bowl and toss with low sodium salt. Let sit till the veggies have released a lot of their liquid.

Separate the veggies from the liquid, reserving the liquid. Place on a tray and place in the freezer for at least a half hour, or until they are partially frozen.

Remove from freezer and let thaw completely.

Combine the thawed veggies, reserved juice, oil and sherry vinegar in a large bowl. Ladle into a blender, working in batches if necessary, and blend on high until quite smooth. Chill for up to 24 hours.

Serve with extra sherry vinegar, olive oil and a sprinkle of chives

242. Munchy Mushroom Soup

Ingredients:
500g boneless chicken breast, sliced
150g button, straw or oyster mushrooms
1 large carrots, sliced
4 red tomatoes, quartered
6 cups low sodium chicken stock
2 stalk lemon grass, sliced into 1 cm pieces
juice from 4-6 limes (add more if you want it sour)
red chillies, chopped

Instructions:
Place the chicken stock in a pot, add lemon grass, and bring to boil over medium heat.

Add the chicken meat, mushrooms, tomatoes, lime juice bring to a boil and simmer for 15 minutes

Add sugar, chillies, carrots and simmer for additional 5 minutes.

Serve while hot.

243. Tempting Tomato Basil Soup

Ingredients:
4 cans whole tomatoes, crushed Note: check for ones without added sugar or salt!
4 cups tomato juice and part low sodium vegetable broth or chicken broth (I use 2 cups tomato juice and 2 cups low sodium chicken broth)
12 or 14 fresh basil leaves
1 cup coconut milk
Low sodium salt and cracked black pepper to taste

Instructions:
Combine tomatoes, juice and/or broth in stockpot. Simmer 30 minutes.

Purée, along with basil leaves, in small batches in a food processor, blender or better yet, a hand-held immersion blender right in the pot.

Return to pot and add coconut milk while stirring over low heat.

244. Healing Chicken/Turkey Vegetable Soup

Ingredients:
Coconut Oil 1 tablespoon
1 medium onion, medium dice
3 medium carrots, medium dice
1 zucchini, medium dice
¼ medium butternut squash, chopped into cubes
12 oz. container of mushrooms, rough dice
2-4 cups shredded chicken
1 tsp. dried thyme
1-2 tsp. dried rosemary + dried basil
½-1 tsp. ground cumin
1 Tbsp. Apple Cider Vinegar
Low sodium salt + pepper
chicken stock
Lemon {optional}

Instructions:
Get a big soup pot on the stove heating on medium with your favorite fat -- I liked coconut oil here because it really warmed up the soup's flavor!

Clean + chop your vegetables and add them in -- literally this is a chop + drop soup. Meaning as you chop just drop it all in and stir occasionally.

Add in as much chicken as you want, I did somewhere between 3-4 cups. I like a lot of chicken in my soup!

Add in your herbs, cumin, apple cider vinegar, low sodium salt + pepper and stir everything together well.

Add in your chicken stock -- I used around half of a batch but honestly just use as much as you want. You want it to cover the vegetables and chicken but after that it's totally up to you how much you add in. And if you don't have enough stock on hand you can always add in a little bit of water!

Stir everything up, cover {with the lid cracked just a little}, and let simmer on low for around an hour or until dinner!

When serving I like to squeeze on a little bit of fresh lemon juice! It makes it even more yummy that it already is!

Notes:
If you want to make this even heartier than it already is, you can add small layer of cauliflower rice to the bottom of your soup bowl, and then ladle the soup on top!

245. Sumptuous Saffron Turkey Cauliflower Soup

Ingredients:
2 tbsp extra virgin olive oil
1 medium onion, chopped (about 1 cup)
2 large garlic cloves, chopped
2 lbs frozen or fresh cauliflower florets
½ tsp low sodium salt
¼ tsp ground black pepper
5 cups of water or vegetable broth
20 saffron threads
Diced Turkey Breast

Instructions:

Sautée onion and garlic in olive oil on a soup pot, over medium heat, until onion is translucent, about 10 minutes.

Add cauliflower florets, low sodium salt and pepper and continue cooking for 10-12 minutes

Add 5 cups of water, bring to a boil and simmer until cauliflower is tender, 20-25 minutes.

Turn off heat. Add saffron, stir and cover. Let the saffron steep for about 20 minutes.

Blend soup in a blender until creamy.

Add Turkey Breast before or after blending

246. Delicious Masala Soup

Ingredients:
1-2 T coconut oil
1 large onion, chopped
2-4 carrots, chopped
3 garlic cloves, chopped
1 head of cauliflower, chopped up
3 cups low sodium chicken broth (or another broth you like)
Diced Turkey Breast
1 cup water
3 tsp dark mustard seeds
2 tsp cumin seeds
1 tsp ground coriander
1 teaspoon ground turmeric
1 tsp low sodium salt
1 T lemon juice
black pepper to taste
crushed red pepper to taste
Optional: chopped cilantro on top

Instructions:
Heat the coconut oil on medium-high and fry the onions, carrots and garlic cloves for about 5+ minutes until they are soft.

Throw in the cauliflower, mustard seeds, cumin, coriander and turmeric.

When the cauliflower is soft, add the chicken broth and water and simmer for 10-15 minutes.

Blend in the food processor until smooth (careful of the splashy hot lava liquid!).

Simmer for another 10 minutes (or until you're ready to eat), add the low sodium salt, pepper, lemon juice and crushed red pepper.

Top with fresh cilantro (I didn't have any, unfortunately) and add turkey breast and EAT.

247. Creamy Chicken Soup

Ingredients:
1/2 cup coconut oil, olive oil, or other oil of choice
2 stalks celery, finely diced
2 medium carrots, finely diced
6 cups low sodium chicken broth
1/2 cup cool water 1 teaspoon dried parsley
1/2 teaspoon dried thyme
1 bay leaf
2 teaspoons low sodium salt 3 cups cooked chicken, cubed
1 1/2 cups coconut milk (1 can full-fat canned or homemade; or pureed cauliflower; see Notes for alternate version)

Instructions:
Place oil in a large soup pot over medium heat. Add the celery and carrots. Cook, stirring occasionally, until soft, 10 to 15 minutes.

Add broth. If using arrowroot, place it and 1/2 cup cool water in a small bowl or jar and whisk or shake to combine. Add to pot along with parsley, thyme, bay leaf, and low sodium salt. Cook, stirring occasionally, until bubbly and thickened (if using arrowroot).

Reduce heat, just enough to maintain a boil, and cook, stirring occasionally for 15 minutes.

Stir in coconut milk (or pureed cauliflower) and chicken and heat through. This is a fairly thick soup; if you like it thinner, add more water, broth, or coconut milk and heat through. Remove bay leaf just before serving. Leftovers may be frozen.

Note:

Alternatively, you can use pureed cauliflower instead of the coconut milk. This version is just as creamy.

To puree the cauliflower, place florets from two medium heads in a pot. Optionally, add a peeled and smashed garlic clove. Add water to cover and about 1/2 tablespoon low sodium salt. Boil 20 minutes or until soft. Drain away water and puree until very smooth using hand blender or other method. Yield is about 4 cups; add the entire amount to the soup.

248. Delicious Lemon-Garlic Soup

Option – add 6 shrimps

Ingredients:
1 tablespoon olive oil
1 tablespoon crushed and chopped fresh garlic
6 cups good-quality low sodium shellfish stock (or mushroom or chicken stock)
2 eggs
1/3 to 1/2 cup fresh lemon juice
1 tablespoon coconut flour for thickening
1/4 teaspoon ground white pepper
chopped fresh cilantro or parsley, if desired

Instructions:

In a 4-quart pot, heat the olive oil over medium-high heat and saute the garlic for 1-2 minutes, or until just fragrant. Do not let the garlic brown.

Reserve 1/2 cup of the stock to mix with the eggs. Pour the remaining 5 1/2 cups of stock into the pot with the garlic. Let the mixture come to a simmer.

In a small bowl, whisk together the eggs, lemon juice, arrowroot, white pepper, and half of a cup of reserved stock. Pour the mixture into the simmering stock and stir until it all thickens--this will only take a few minutes.

Serve the soup hot, sprinkled with fresh cilantro or parsley.

249. Turkey Squash Soup

Ingredients:
1 large acorn squash
1/2 teaspoon olive oil
low sodium salt and pepper to taste
2 cups chicken or vegetable stock
1/4 cup coconut milk
1-2 turkey breasts shredded
3/4 teaspoon ground ginger
1 tablespoon coconut aminos
Pinch or two of cayenne pepper
Pomegranate seeds and/or sliced almonds, for serving

Instructions:
Preheat the oven to 400. Cut the acorn squash in half and scoop out the seeds and pulp. Brush each half with about 1/4 teaspoon olive oil and sprinkle with low sodium salt and pepper. Place in a foil-lined baking pan and roast, cut sides up, until fork tender (about an hour).

When the squash is cool enough to handle, scoop out the flesh and place it in a medium saucepan, or in a blender if you don't have an immersion blender. Add the remaining ingredients and process with an immersion blender (or regular blender) until smooth. Place the saucepan over medium heat and cook, stirring often, until heated through. Serve hot or warm, with pomegranate seeds and/or sliced almonds.

250. Roasted Winter Vegetable Turkey Soup

Ingredients:
2 large onions, cut into eighths
2 large sweet potatoes, peeled and cut into 1 inch dice
2 lbs of carrots, peeled and cut into 2 inch dice
1 head (yes head) of garlic, cloves peeled
4 tbsp coconut oil
low sodium salt and pepper to taste
2 cups low sodium chicken stock
1-2 turkey breasts

Instructions:
Preheat the oven to 425 degrees F.

Distribute the onions, garlic, sweet potatoes and carrots evenly on a sheet tray- it will likely require two trays.

Top the vegetables with coconut oil. You can melt the oil ahead of time if it is solid, or wait until it melts in the oven and then stir it around. Season GENEROUSLY with low sodium salt and pepper.

Roast for 25-35 minutes until vegetables are tender, flipping halfway through cooking.

When the veggies have roasted, transfer them into a large pot on the stove top. Add just enough chicken stock to cover the veggies by 1 inch.

Put the lid on and bring the liquid to a boil. Reduce the heat and simmer with the lid cracked for 10 minutes.

Now you get to puree your soup! You can do this in a blender, but do it in small batches so that it doesn't explode on you. But I love to use my immersion blender. It's convenient and you don't have to mess with all of the transferring and what not.

Taste and season with low sodium salt and pepper if needed.

Spoon it up and eat it as is, or stir in a bit of coconut cream add turkey- Enjoy!

251. Jam and 'Cream' Cupcakes

cupcakes
1/2 cup coconut flour, sifted
1/4 cup arrowroot (tapioca flour), sifted
4 eggs
5 drops stevia liquid (May need a few more – please taste test)
3 tablespoons coconut oil
1 cup full fat coconut cream
1/2 teaspoon concentrated natural vanilla extract
pinch of low sodium salt
1 teaspoon baking powder
sugar free strawberry jam*
1 punnet of strawberries (250 grams or approximately 1 heaped cup of chopped strawberries)
2 tablespoons chia seeds
2 drops stevia
Place the ingredients into blender or food processor and blend until smooth and well combined. Pour / spoon the mixture into a container and place in the fridge to thicken.
'cream'*
1 cup raw macadamias
1/2 teaspoon concentrated natural vanilla extract
pinch of low sodium salt

Instructions
1. Place the ingredients into your blender or food processor and blend at high speed until you have a lovely, smooth macadamia butter. I leave this at room temperature as I find it easier to work with when assembling the cupcakes. After that I store the remaining butter in the fridge.
2. Preheat your oven to 175 degrees Celsius or 350 degrees Fahrenheit.
3. Line nine holes of a standard muffin tray with cupcake cases.
4. In a medium sized bowl beat together your stevia and coconut oil. Add in the eggs, coconut cream and vanilla. 5. Add the flours and when smooth and well combined gently add the salt and baking powder.
6. Spoon the mixture evenly into your nine cases.
7. Bake for 25 minutes.
8. Allow to cool slightly before moving from the tray to a cooling rack.
9. Leave the cakes to cool completely before using a small, sharp knife to remove the tops of the cupcakes and create a small indent in the cake. Fill the cake with a teaspoon of jam and a teaspoon of 'cream' (macadamia butter).
10. Gently place the cupcake 'lid' back on top.
11. Eat and enjoy!!!

252. Delicious Yellow Cupcake Recipe

Ingredients
Cake
½ cup of sifted Organic coconut flour
5 large eggs
⅓ cup of butter or ghee or coconut oil
1 teaspoon vanilla
5 drops stevia liquid (May need a few more – please taste test)
1 cup of applesauce
1 teaspoon baking powder
1 teaspoon baking soda

Instructions:
Combine the coconut flour, baking powder and baking soda in a bowl and blend.
Add in all the liquid ingredients; mix well with a spoon.
Pour into the cupcake tins and bake at 350 degrees for 20 minutes.
Frost and enjoy!

253. Perfect Pear & Nutmeg Cupcakes

Ingredients
2 ripe pears, peeled, de-cored and chopped into small pieces
1 tsp nutmeg
1 tbsp water
1/4 cup coconut flour
2 large eggs
1/4 cup coconut oil or melted butter
5 drops stevia liquid (May need a few more – please taste test)
1/4 tsp baking powder

Instructions
Add the pear, water, 5 drops stevia and 1/2 tsp of nutmeg to a saucepan. Let the mixture simmer over a medium heat until the pears soften (about 15 mins). Either mash with a hand-masher or transfer to a blender and puree. Set aside to cool.

Sieve the coconut flour, the remaining tsp of nutmeg and baking powder into a mixing bowl. In a separate bowl, beat the eggs, coconut oil/butter and stevia together.

If the pear puree is cool, stir it into the eggs.

Gradually add the wet ingredients to the dry and stir until it forms a semi-runny batter.

Spoon into a muffin tray (it should make 6 muffins). Bake at 375 for 12-15 mins.

254. Xmas Chocolate Chip Cupcakes

Ingredients
1/2 c Coconut Flour
5 Eggs
2 Egg Whites
1/2 c Cashew Butter (or coconut oil for nut free)
1/2 t low sodium Salt
1/2 t Baking Soda
1/2 t Gluten Free Baking Powder
5 drops stevia liquid (May need a few more – please taste test)
3/4 c Egg Nog
1/4 t Vanilla
1/2 t Nutmeg
1 c Chocolate Chips
Vanilla Frosting
1 c coconut oil
2 T Canned Coconut Milk
1 t Vanilla

Instructions
Whisk together the dry ingredients.
Beat the eggs, whites, egg nog, butter, vanilla, and stevia. By 1/2 cup-fulls, add the dry mixture and whisk until smooth. Fold in the chocolate chips.
Preheat the oven to 350 degrees. Fill lined muffin tins 1/2 full with batter. Bake for 25-30 minutes, or until a toothpick.
If you want to do a loaf instead, bake in a loaf pan, same temp, for 50-55 mins.
For the frosting, beat all the ingredients till light and fluffy!

Paleo Diet Recipes 365 Days Of Anti-Inflammatory Recipes
By Mercedes Del Rey

255. Boston Cream Pie Cupcake Bonanza

Vanilla Cream
Ingredients:
2 organic cage-free egg yolks
5 drops stevia liquid (May need a few more – please taste test)
2 tablespoons coconut palm sugar
2 tablespoons plus 1/2 teaspoon arrowroot starch/flour
pinch of pink low of sodium salt
1 cup canned coconut cream/milk, full fat, room temperature
1/2 teaspoon vanilla

Cupcakes
Ingredients:
1 & 1/2 cups fine blanched almond flour
1 & 1/2 teaspoons baking powder
1/2 teaspoon pink low sodium salt
1/2 cup canned coconut cream/milk, full fat, room temperature
6 tablespoons unsalted grass-fed butter, plus more for greasing
3 organic cage-free eggs
1 cup coconut palm sugar
1 teaspoon vanilla

Chocolate Ganache
Ingredients:
1 cup Enjoy Life Mini Chocolate Chips
1/4 cup canned coconut cream/milk, full fat, room temperature
4 tablespoons unsalted grass-fed butter
1 teaspoon vanilla

Directions:
1. Start by making the Vanilla Cream. In a small bowl whisk egg yolks together until smooth, set aside. In a medium saucepan combine stevia, coconut palm sugar, arrowroot, and salt and stir over medium heat. Add milk in a slow steady stream. Stir and let cook until the mixture begins to boil and thicken, about 5 minutes.
2. Pour 1/3 of the milk mixture into the yolks and stir together with a whisk until combined. Then pour back into the saucepan with the rest of the milk mixture and cook over medium heat, stirring often, until thick, about 3 minutes. Now stir in the vanilla.
3. Use a fine sieve to pour the vanilla mixture through into a small bowl. Cover it with plastic wrap and press the wrap down directly on to the surface of the cream. Refrigerate until very cold, an hour at least. While you wait prepare your cupcakes and chocolate ganache.
4. Preheat oven to 350. Grease a mini cupcake pan very liberally with butter. In a large bowl combine almond flour, baking powder and salt, use a fork to stir together. Warm coconut cream/milk and butter in a saucepan over low heat.

5. In a separate large bowl, whisk together eggs and coconut palm sugar. Then fold in the dry mixture.

6. Bring the coconut cream/milk and butter mixture to a boil. Add this mixture to the batter and whisk until smooth. Now stir in the vanilla. Pour batter into a Ziploc bag, cut a small hole in the corner. Transfer batter to prepared pan, filling to the top. Bake for 10-12 minutes or until a toothpick comes out clean. While you are waiting for the cupcakes to cool, go ahead and make your chocolate ganache.

7. Using the double boiler method melt together the chocolate, coconut cream/milk and butter. Once melted and combined stir in the vanilla. Transfer ganache to a Ziploc bag once it's cool enough, and cut a small hole in the corner tip.

8. Once your cupcakes are cool, remove two from the pan at a time. Squeeze a layer of vanilla cream over the top of one cupcake and then flip the other one upside down and use it to sandwich the two together. Then pour your chocolate ganache over the top and enjoy!

Notes:

You may have noticed above it says Coconut Cream or Coconut Milk. Coconut Cream can be found at health food stores like Sprouts or Whole Foods next to the regular coconut milk. I prefer it because it's a little thicker than normal coconut milk, so if you can find it use it, if not coconut milk will work just fine.

256. Vanilla Bean Cupcakes with Mocha Buttercream

Ingredients
(makes 5-6 cupcakes):
For the cupcakes
1/4 cup coconut flour, sifted
1/4 teaspoon low sodium salt
1/8 teaspoon baking soda
Seeds scraped from half a vanilla bean
1/2 teaspoon vanilla extract
3 large eggs
1/4 cup coconut oil
5 drops stevia liquid (May need a few more – please taste test)

Insytructions
Preheat the oven to 350 and line a muffin tin with paper liners. Whisk together the coconut flour, salt, and baking soda in a medium bowl. Add the vanilla bean seeds, and mix together with your fingers, pinching the mixture to evenly distribute the vanilla seeds. In a small bowl, whisk together the vanilla extract, eggs, coconut oil, and stevia. Add the wet ingredients to the dry and whisk well, or beat with a hand mixer, until very smooth. Pour the batter into the cupcake cups and bake for 15-20 minutes, or until a toothpick comes out clean.

For the frosting:
8 tablespoons 1 stick) unsalted butter, at room temperature
5 drops stevia liquid (May need a few more – please taste test)
1 tablespoon cocoa
Tiny pinch of low sodium salt
1/4 teaspoon vanilla extract
1/4 teaspoon finely ground coffee
Coffee beans for garnish

Using a hand mixer, beat the butter until very smooth. Add the remaining ingredients and beat until incorporated. If your frosting does not seem stiff enough, refrigerate for a little while, then beat again. Once the cupcakes are completely cool, pipe or spread on the frosting (I used a Wilton 1M tip). Top with a coffee bean if desired.

257. Meaty Meatloaf Cupcakes

Ingredients
1.5-2 pounds of ground beef (grass-fed if possible)
3 eggs
¼ cup almond flour (or enough to thicken- this will depend partially on the fat content of the meat and the texture of the almond flour)
1 teaspoon dried basil
1 teaspoon garlic powder
1 medium onion
2 tablespoons worcestershire sauce
Salt and pepper to taste
5-6 sweet potatoes
¼ cup butter or coconut oil
1 teaspoon low sodium Salt

Instructions
Preheat the oven to 375 degrees
Finely dice the onion or puree in a blender or food processor.
In a large bowl, combine the meat, eggs, flour, basil, garlic powder, pureed onion, Worcestershire sauce, and salt and pepper and mix by hand until incorporated.
Grease a muffin tin with coconut oil or butter and evenly divide the mixture into the muffin tins to make 2-3 meat "muffins" per person. If you don't have a muffin tin, you can just press the mixture into the bottom of an 8x8 or 9x13 baking dish.
Put into oven on middle rack, and put a baking sheet with a rim under it, in case the oil from the meat happens to spill over (should only happen with fattier meats if at all)
For sweet potatoes: if they are small enough, you can put them into the oven at the same time, if not you can peel, cube and boil them until soft.
When meat is almost done, make sure sweet potatoes are cooked by whichever method you prefer, and drain the water if you boiled them.
Mix with butter and salt or pepper if desired and mash by hand or with an immersion blender.
Remove meat "muffins" from the oven when they are cooked through and remove from tin. Top each with a dollop of the mashed sweet potatoes to make it look like a cupcake.

258. Gushing Guava Cupcakes with Whipped Guava Frosting

Ingredients
For the Cake
¾ cup (120g) of Coconut Flour
¾ cup (96g) of Tapioca Flour
¾ cup of Light Olive Oil
6 Tablespoons (85g) of Granulated Sugar or Coconut Sugar
5 drops stevia liquid (May need a few more – please taste test)
½ cup of Concentrated Guava Puree ('applesauce thick')
6 Eggs
1 teaspoon of Lime Juice
1½ teaspoon of Cream of Tartar
¾ teaspoon of Baking Soda
½ teaspoon of low sodium Salt
For the Whipped Guava Frosting
¾ cup of room temperature coconut oil
6 Tablespoons of Concentrated Guava Puree ('applesauce thick')
5 drops stevia liquid (May need a few more – please taste test)
½ cup of Arrowroot Starch, sifted
1 teaspoon of Lime
Pinch of low sodium Salt

Instructions
For the Cake
You may have to boil the guava puree until applesauce thick. I used Goya brand and let it boil for about 10 minutes.
Preheat oven to 350F. We will drop the temperature to 325F to bake. Line the muffin tin with cupcake liners.
Separate the eggs into egg yolks and egg whites.
Combine the egg whites and cream of tartar and beat with a whisk attachment on high speed. Place the whites in a bowl and set aside, or store in the refrigerator while preparing the rest of the ingredients.
Combine the olive oil, egg yolks, stevia, lime juice, and guava puree in the mixing bowl and beat on high speed for about 30 seconds.
Sift together the coconut flour, tapioca flour, baking soda, sugar, and salt to make the dry flour mixture.
Add half of the dry flour mixture to the wet mixture and whip until the flours absorb and the batter becomes fluffy. Scrape the sides with a spatula to incorporate.
Add the rest of the dry flour mixture and beat on high speed with the whisk until combined and fluffy.
Scoop in a heaping of the egg white meringue and hand mix into the batter. Gently fold in the rest of the meringue until combined.
Portion the batter into each cake pan and place tin in the oven centered.

Paleo Diet Recipes 365 Days Of Anti-Inflammatory Recipes
By Mercedes Del Rey

Reduce the temperature to 325F and for 25-30 minutes until an inserted toothpick comes out clean.
This method will give a nice dome to the cupcakes and prevent over browning of the stevia.
Let cool to room temperature or colder before frosting.
For the Frosting
Chill the beaters and mixing bowl in the freezer for about 15 minutes.
Combine the raw stevia and guava puree in a cup until it forms a thicker syrup.
Whip the coconut shortening and optionally the cream cheese.
Add the arrowroot starch and salt and whip.
While mixing on medium speed, pour the guava mixture slowly. Whip until pink and pretty.
Add more stevia to taste if you like.
Dollop onto a cooled cupcake and enjoy!

259. Blushing Blueberry Muffin Recipe

Ingredients
2 1/2 cups almond flour
1 Tablespoon coconut flour
1/4 teaspoon low sodium salt
1/2 teaspoon baking soda
1 Tablespoon vanilla
1/4 cup coconut oil
5 drops stevia liquid (May need a few more – please taste test)
1/4 cup coconut milk*
2 eggs
1 cup fresh or frozen blueberries
2-3 Tablespoons cinnamon

Instructions
Preheat oven to 350. Line a 12 count muffin tin and lightly oil with coconut oil.
In a mixing bowl combine almond flour, coconut flour, salt, and baking soda and stir to combine.
Pour in coconut oil, eggs, stevia, coconut milk, and vanilla; mix well.
Fold in blueberries and add cinnamon.
Distribute into muffin tin. Sprinkle with additional cinnamon.
Bake for 22-25 minutes. Allow to cool and enjoy!

Notes
*Coconut milk can come in different textures depending on the brand you use. If you use a thicker brand like THAI, then use 1/8 cup of coconut milk and 4 Tablespoons of water. If your coconut milk is thinner, stick to the 1/4 cup of coconut milk.

260. Healthy Carrot Ginger Muffins

Ingredients:
2 cups blanched almond flour
½ teaspoon low sodium salt
1 teaspoon baking soda
½ tsp allspice
½ tsp powdered ginger
a pinch of clove
½ cup shredded coconut shreds, unsweetened
3 eggs, preferably pastured
½ cup coconut oil, melted
5 drops stevia liquid (May need a few more – please taste test)
1-2 Tbs grated fresh ginger
1 cup grated carrot
3/4 cup raisins, soaked in water for 15 minutes and drained

Instructions:
In a large bowl, combine almond flour, salt, baking soda, spices, and coconut shreds
In a smaller bowl whisk together eggs, oil, and syrup. Add fresh ginger, grated carrot, and raisins.
Stir wet ingredients into dry
Spoon batter into paper-lined muffin tins
Bake at 350° for 18-20 minutes for mini muffins OR 24-26 minutes for regular muffins.
Cool and serve.

261. Pecan Muffins

(makes 12)

Ingredients

1/3 cup coconut flour
1/4 cup butter, melted
3 large eggs
1/3 cup chopped pecans
1/4 tsp baking powder
stevia drops to taste

Instructions

Whisk together the butter, eggs and molasses.

Sieve the coconut flour and baking powder into a large mixing bowl.

Gradually add the wet ingredients to the dry, stirring until it forms a thick, runny Fold in the pecans.

Spoon about a tbsp into small (I used 4cm) muffin cups. It should stretch to 12. Bake at 350 for 10-12 minutes.

262. Temptingly Perfect Plantain Drop

Ingredients
3 tablespoons coconut oil
2 brown plantains (they must be brown)
1 tsp stevia
¼ cup coconut oil, melted
3 eggs
1 tablespoon canned coconut milk
3 tablespoons coconut flour
1-2 teaspoons cinnamon (I used 2 because I love cinnamon)
1 teaspoon baking powder
A pinch of low sodium salt

Instructions
1. Preheat oven to 350 degrees.
2. Cut the ends off of the plantains, then use your knife to cut them in half lengthwise and then peel the skin off, cutting off any excess skin that sticks to the plantains. The browner the plantains are, the sweeter they will be and the easier the skin is to take off.
3. Now place a large skillet over medium-high heat, add 3 tablespoons of coconut oil to heat up, then add the halved plantains to the skillet. Cook on both sides for about 3-4 minutes until browned, making sure not to burn them.
4. Once the plantains are done cooking, add them to the food processor and puree until they begin to clump together.
5. Then add the stevia, coconut oil, eggs, and coconut milk and puree until smooth. No clumps should be present at this point.
6. Now add coconut flour, cinnamon, baking powder, and salt to the food processor and puree one more time to combine everything well.
7. Now line a baking sheet with parchment paper and grab an ice cream scoop to help form perfect sized biscuits.
8. Scoop the batter out and plop each biscuit on the baking sheet about 1 inch away from each other. My batter made 8 biscuits.
9. Place in oven and bake for 20-25 minutes until slightly brown and completely cooked through.
10. Let cool. These babies are hot and need to settle afterwards.

263. Sweety Potato Muffins

Ingredients
1/2 c Coconut Flour
6 Eggs
2 t Vanilla
1 t low sodium Salt
1 t Baking Soda
2 t Cinnamon
1/2 c Ground Flax
2 Sweet Potatoes or Yams, baked and mashed (discard skins)
1 c Raisins or Chocolate Chips (optional)

Instructions:
Whisk together all the dry ingredients. Beat the eggs and add dry mix by spoonfuls until well blended. Add the mashed sweet potatoes.
Spoon batter into lined muffin cups. Bake at 350 degrees for 30-35 minutes.
Enjoy!

264. Zesty Zucchini Muffins

Ingredients
3/4 C applesauce
5 drops stevia liquid (May need a few more – please taste test)
1/4 C coconut oil, melted
3 eggs
1 Tbsp vanilla
2 C almond flour
1 1/2 tsp baking soda
1 C zucchini, shredded
3/4 C raisin

Instructions
With electric or stand mixer, beat applesauce, stevia and oil
Add eggs and vanilla and mix until combined
Slowly mix in almond flour and soda, then beat until batter forms
Fold in zucchini and raisins
Bake at 350 degrees for 25 minutes, makes 15 muffins

265. Cozy Coconut Flour Muffins

Ingredients
1/2 cup coconut flour
6 eggs, at room temperature (that's important)
¼ cup almond milk
2 tsp stevia
6 Tbs. coconut oil
2 Tbsp coconut milk at room temperature
2 tsp. vanilla extract
1/4 tsp. baking soda
1 tsp. apple cider vinegar

Instructions
Preheat the oven to 350 degrees and prepare a muffin tin with 8 liners (I like unbleached parchment paper baking cups).
Combine the coconut flour and eggs until smooth. Add the remaining ingredients and stir well.
Divide evenly between the muffin tins. Bake until golden and a toothpick comes out clean, about 20 minutes.
Cool completely.

**Makes 8 cupcakes. Feel free to double the recipe if you want more cupcakes! These last in an airtight container for a few days at room temperature. They also freeze really well!

266. Lemon Mousse Mouthwatering Cupcakes

Ingredients
1/2 cup coconut flour
6 eggs, at room temperature (that's important)
6 Tbs. milk
2 tsp stevia
6 Tbs. coconut oil
2 Tbs. coconut milk at room temperature
1 tsp. vanilla extract
1/2 tsp. ground cardamom
1/4 tsp. baking soda
1/2 tsp. apple cider vinegar

Instructions
Preheat the oven to 350 degrees and prepare a muffin tin with 8 liners (I like unbleached parchment paper baking cups).
Combine the coconut flour and eggs until smooth. Add the remaining ingredients and stir well.
Divide evenly between the muffin tins. Bake until golden and a toothpick comes out clean, about 20 minutes.
Cool completely and frost with the lemon mousse.
Makes 8 cupcakes. Feel free to double the recipe if you want more cupcakes!

Lemon Mousse Frosting

Ingredients
3/4 cup stevia-sweetened lemon curd (recipe below)
1 cup coconut milk
1 Tbs. light coconut milk
1 tsp stevia
Pinch of low sodium salt to taste

Instructions
First, make the stevia-sweetened lemon curd, by simply whisking the whole eggs, yolks and 1tsp stevia in a saucepan until smooth, then place pan over a low heat. Add the coconut oil, juice and zest and whisk continuously until thickened. Strain through a sieve. Lemon curd keeps, covered, in the fridge for 2 weeks. Chill until thickened and cold before using it.
In a small saucepan, whisk together the coconut milk and gelatin. Let it sit for 10 minutes. Then turn the heat on medium and whisk until the gelatin dissolves. Pour into a bowl and refrigerate until set, about 4 hours.
In a food processor, blend together the set coconut milk and the lemon curd until smooth. Add stevia to taste and a small pinch of low sodium salt.

267. Sexy Savory Muffins

Ingredients
½ cup coconut flour
1 tsp baking soda
½-1 tsp low sodium salt
¼ cup coconut oil
½ cup + 2 tbsp coconut milk
4 pastured eggs
1 tsp apple cider vinegar
1 tsp garlic powder
½ tsp each of rosemary, thyme, sage

Instructions

1. Pre-heat the oven to 350°. Melt the coconut oil and combine with remaining muffin ingredients in a food procssor or bowl, mix well.
2. Place batter in a muffine tin lined with muffin liners. The muffins will raise a small amount, so you can fill the muffin liner about ¾ full–almost to the top. Bake for about 20-30 minutes or until a toothpick inserted comes out clean and the tops are slightly browned.
3. Let it cool and slice in small squares.

268. Molten Lava Chocolate Cupcake

Ingredients:
4 oz Semi-Sweet or Bittersweet chocolate
½ tsp Vanilla Extract
1/8 tsp Salt
5 drops stevia liquid (May need a few more – please taste test)
1 tsp Coconut Flour
2 tsp Cacao Powder
2 eggs
4 Tbsp extra virgin coconut oil (plus a little more for greasing the ramekins)

Instructions:
1. Preheat oven to 375F. Grease four 6oz ramekins with coconut oil.
2. In a 4 cup measuring cup or medium microwave-safe bowl, melt chocolate and coconut oil in the microwave on low power. Stir until smooth and let cool.
3. In a small bowl, beat eggs, vanilla, salt and sugar with a hand mixer until light and frothy, about five minutes (this can seem like an eternity with a hand mixer, but hang in there because it's worth it!).
4. Pour egg mixture over chocolate. Sift cocoa and coconut flour over the top. Then gently fold all the ingredients together.
5. Pour batter into prepared ramekins (they should be filled to within ½" of the top). Place the ramekins on a baking sheet and place in the oven (you can chill the ramekins for a few hours if you want to make them ahead of time, just make sure you bring them back to room temperature before baking). Bake for 11-12 minutes.
6. Remove from oven and serve immediately. Enjoy!

269. Party Carrot Cupcakes

Ingredients
Wet
3 eggs
6 tablespoon non-dairy milk
6 tablespoon extra virgin coconut oil, melted
6 tablespoon carrot juice
5½ tablespoon egg whites
30 drops liquid stevia*see note
¾ teaspoon pure vanilla extract
Dry
6 tablespoon coconut flour
1 teaspoon baking powder
¼ teaspoon low sodium salt
pinch ground cinnamon

Instructions
Preheat oven to 350F and line 12 muffin tins with medium-sized paper liners.
Place eggs and egg white in blender and beat well, about 30 seconds. My magic bullet worked great for this!
Pour in carrot juice, milk, coconut oil, stevia and vanilla. Blend quickly to mix.
Drop in dry ingredients and mix for about 10 seconds. The batter should be slightly thicker than pancake batter.
Pour into prepared muffin tins and bake for 25-30 minutes or until inserted toothpick comes out clean. Mine took 26 minutes. Remove from pan and allow to cool on cooling rack for at least 1 hour before applying buttercream.

270. Cinnamon Chocolate Chip Muffins

Ingredients
Muffins
6 large eggs
5 drops stevia liquid (May need a few more – please taste test)
1 teaspoon vanilla extract
8 tablespoons (1 stick) unsalted butter, melted
3/4 cup coconut flour
1 tablespoon ground cinnamon
2 teaspoons baking powder
1 teaspoon baking soda
small pinch low sodium salt

Instructions
Muffins
Preheat oven to 375 fahrenheit and adjust rack to middle position
Line with muffin liners
Whisk eggs, stevia, vanilla, butter, and applesauce in a large mixing bowl or use a stand mixer
Sift coconut flour, cinnamon, baking powder, baking soda, and salt over a medium bowl
Add dry ingredients to wet ingredients and until well blended
Fold in chocolate chips ensuring an even distribution throughout your batter
Spoon batter into muffin cups and bake for 16-18 minutes, or until a toothpick in the center comes out clean
Remove the muffins from the oven and let cool
Once cool you can head below and make the frosting to go with them
Notes
*You can not let Coconut flour sit long, as soon as you mix this batter, ensure you put it right into the oven *If you want chocolate muffins, you can add between 1/4 - 1/2 cup of cocoa powder to your taste liking *You can store these in an airtight container for 3 days *You can substitute the butter with Coconut Oil but I haven't tested it and 8 tablespoons would probably be too oily. If you do test it, start with half and please let me know how it worked.

271. Strawberry Shortcake Cupcakes

Ingredients:
2½ cups blanched almond flour
¾ teaspoon baking soda
¼ teaspoon low sodium salt
5 drops stevia liquid (May need a few more – please taste test)
⅓ cup coconut oil, melted
4 large eggs, room temperature
1 tablespoon lemon juice
2 teaspoons vanilla extract
½ teaspoon lemon zest
½ cup finely chopped strawberries
Frosting
2 egg whites, room temperature
5 drops stevia liquid (May need a few more – please taste test)
¼ teaspoon lemon juice or vinegar
1½ tablespoons strawberry preserves (freshly pureed strawberries will work too)

Instructions:
Preheat the oven to 325 degrees F.
Line a standard muffin tin with baking cups.
Combine the stevia, coconut oil, eggs, lemon juice, vanilla, and lemon zest in the jar of a blender. Puree on medium speed for 20 seconds or until frothy and smooth.
Add the dry ingredients and blend on high for 30-45 seconds. The batter should be very smooth and contain no lumps. If needed, scrape down the sides with a spatula and blend again for a few seconds until all of the dry mixture is incorporated.
Gently fold the chopped strawberries in by hand. Divide the batter evenly into the muffin tin, filling about ¾ of the way full.
Bake for 16-18 minutes, until a toothpick can be inserted into the middle and comes out clean.
Let the cupcakes cool completely on the counter before frosting.
Frosting
Once the cupcakes have cooled, make your Italian meringue.
Bring your stevia to a boil in a saucepan over medium-high heat.
Meanwhile, beat the egg whites and lemon juice until frothy and you can just begin to see trail marks from your beaters. When you lift out the beaters, you should see soft peaks.
With the beaters or mixer running, slowly pour in the boiling stevia in a steady stream. Continue beating for 6-8 minutes, until the meringue is cool to the touch.
Gently fold in the strawberry preserves. Put the frosting into a piping bag for a pretty design, or spread onto cupcakes with a knife.
Tips

For easier separation, separate the whites from the yolks when they are cold.
Meringue will not stiffen if you use a dirty bowl (usually because of leftover oil) or let any of the yolk get in with the whites
Over beating will cause the meringue to fall. Stop once you can lift the beaters out and see stiff peaks.
The frosting needs to be piped immediately and is best served immediately as well. Once it's on the cupcakes though, it will hold up in the refrigerator for 24 hours.

272. Thin Mint Mini Cupcakes

Ingredients
For the Cupcakes
1/4 cup coconut flour
1/4 cup organic cocoa powder
4 large eggs (at room temperature)
1/4 cup coconut oil
5 drops stevia liquid (May need a few more – please taste test)
1/4 tsp baking soda
1 tsp lemon juice
Pinch of low sodium salt
1/4 tsp mint extract
6 Tbsp chopped dark chocolate or dairy free chocolate chips (for Paleo)

For the frosting:
2/3 cup powdered sweetener or coconut sugar, powdered for Paleo
2 ripe avocado
1/2 cup coconut milk
1/4 tsp mint extract

Instructions
Preheat oven to 350 F
Combine the coconut flour, cocoa powder, sweetener (if granular), baking soda, and low sodium salt.
In a separate bowl, combine the eggs, coconut oil, and lemon juice (and stevia if using).
Add the dry ingredients to the wet and mix to combine.
Line a mini muffin tin with 24 cupcake liners.
Fill cupcake liners evenly with the batter and bake for 13-15 minutes or until cooked through.
Allow to cool before topping with the icing.
Pipe on the frosting (directions below) onto each cupcake and serve.
For the frosting
Place the meat of the avocados in a blender and mix until completely smooth.
Add the sweetener, coconut milk, and mint extract. Mix until thoroughly incorporated.
Notes
Total Carb Count: 3.1 g (for 1 mini cupcake plus the carbs for the sweetener used)
Net Carb Count: 1.2 g net carbs (for 1 mini cupcake plus the carbs for the sweetener used)
*Note carb counts are estimated based on the products I used. Check nutrition labels for accurate carb counts and gluten information.

273. Lemon-Coconut Petit Fours

Ingredients
For the Cake
1/2 cup coconut flour
1/2 cup coconut milk
3 eggs, separated
3/4 cup soaked dates in 3 tbsp hot water
1/2 tsp vanilla
1/2 tsp baking soda
1/4 tsp low sodium salt
1 tsp lemon rind

Frosting
2/3 cup coconut cream (from the top of a can of coconut milk)
2 tbsp almond milk
1 tbsp Stevia
3 tsp lemon juice
¼ cup coconut oil, room temperature

Instructions
Put dates in a heat safe bowl or container and pour 3 tbsp boiling water over them and let soak for about 15 minutes. You can chop the dates before soaking to speed up the process, but it's not necessary. Separate the eggs with yolks in one bowl and whites in one large stainless steel, glass or ceramic bowl. When you go to whip the egg whites, it helps if they are at room temperature.
Once dates have soaked put them in a food processor along with remaining water and mix until you have a paste-like consistency. Add coconut flour, milk, egg yolks, vanilla, baking soda, salt and lemon rind and mix.
Whip the egg whites until foamy and stiff peaks form. This is much easier if you have a stand mixer with the whisk attachment or a hand mixer. It is possible to do it by hand, but takes time.
Gently fold egg whites into the batter. Grease a standard sized loaf pan. Put batter in pan and even out the top with a spatula or spoon.
Bake in a 350° oven for 20-30 minutes or when a toothpick inserted comes out clean.

For the frosting
Coconut cream can be purchased in cans or you can skim the cream of the top of cans of coconut milk, however you may have to use multiple cans of coconut milk. Put coconut cream in a bowl and whisk for a few minutes to make it lighter and creamier.
Add coconut oil, milk, stevia and lemon juice and whisk until fully incorporated.

Allow the cake to cool completely before frosting. Once the cake has cooled, cut small squares or circles out of the cake and skim some cake off of the top with a knife to make it even. There will be leftover scraps, but they make a great snack!

Cut the squares in half and frost the middle. You can use the prepared frosting, but it will be very thin. Drizzle the prepared frosting over the small cake squares and use a spatula or knife to frost the sides evenly. Once you've frosted each petit fours, refrigerate to allow the frosting to harden. Top with a bit of lemon rind.

274. Blushing Blueberry Cupcakes

Ingredients:
1/2 cup almond flour
1/2 cup coconut flour
1/2 cup hazelnut flour
1 tbsp coconut sugar
1 tsp baking soda
¼ tsp low sodium salt
3 eggs
3 tbsp unsweetened almond milk
5 drops stevia liquid (May need a few more – please taste test)
1 tsp vanilla extract
½ cup blueberries

Instructions
Preheat oven to 350°.
Combine dry ingredients (both flours, sugar, baking soda, and salt) into a bowl and mix.
In a separate bowl, whisk eggs together; add milk, stevia and vanilla and stir.
Fold wet ingredients into dry ingredients.
Stir in the blueberries by hand.
Line muffin tin with muffin liners and spray each one with a bit of nonstick spray (optional but recommended).
Pour batter evenly to your cupcake tray
Bake for 10-15 minutes or until batter is no longer in liquid form.
Drizzle with extra stevia if desired.
Enjoy!

275. Delicious Morning Cupcakes

Ingredients
1/3 cup mashed sweet potato
3 eggs
¼ 5 drops stevia liquid (May need a few more – please taste test)
1 teaspoon pure vanilla extract
1 cup grated carrot (1 large)
1 cup grated apple (½ large Fugi)
2 teaspoons fresh ginger, peeled and grated, optional
2 cups blanched almond flour
1 cup unsweetened shredded coconut (or flaked coconut)
2/3 cup raisins
2/3 cup raw walnuts, chopped
2 teaspoons ground cinnamon
1 teaspoon baking powder
¼ teaspoon baking soda
½ teaspoon low sodium salt

Instructions
Preheat the oven to 350 degrees F and line a 12-cupcake tray with baking cups.
Whisk together the mashed sweet potato, eggs, stevia, grated carrot, apple, and ginger until well-combined (wet ingredients).
In a seperate mixing bowl, stir together the almond flour, raisins, walnuts, cinnamon, baking powder, baking soda, and salt (dry ingredients).
Pour the dry mixture into the bowl with the wet mixture and stir well until a thick batter forms.
using an ice cream scoop or small measuring cup, scoop batter into the lined muffin tray, filling the cups 3/4 of the way up.
Place cupcake tray on the center rack in the preheated oven and bake for 30 to 35 minutes, until cupcake test clean when poked with a toothpick.
Allow cupcakes to cool at least 20 minutes before mowing them down < - if you try to eat the cupcakes before letting them cool, they will stick to the cupcake cups like whoa.

276. Cheerful Coffee Cupcake

Cupcake Ingredients:
6 eggs
1/4 cup ghee
1/4 cup coconut flour
1/4 cup water chestnut flour 2 Tbsp grade B stevia 2 Tbsp vanilla
5 drops stevia liquid (May need a few more – please taste test)
1/4 tsp low sodium salt
1/2 tsp cinnamon

Topping Ingredients:
1/2 cup pecans (chopped)
5 drops stevia liquid (May need a few more – please taste test)
4 Tbsp ghee
2 Tbsp almond flour
1 tsp cinnamon
1/8 tsp low sodium salt

Instructions
Preheat oven to 350 degrees.
Put eggs in a large mixing bowl and mix thoroughly with an immersion blender until frothy.
Add remaining ingredients and mix well.
Fill muffin pan evenly (should make 1 dozen).
Place in oven and set timer for 20 minutes.
Now combine ingredients for the topping in a separate bowl.
At the 20 minute mark take out the muffins and add the topping evenly between all the muffins.
Put them back in the oven for another 10 minutes.
Broil for an additional 2 minutes and remove quickly.
Let cool.
Enjoy with a hot cup of coffee! Ok, I guess I'll let you do tea if you insist

277. Luscious Lemon Poppy Seed Cupcake

Ingredients
1 1/4 cup almond flour
2 tbs coconut flour
1 tbs poppy seeds
1 tsp baking soda
1 tsp baking powder
1/4 tsp low sodium salt
5 drops stevia liquid (May need a few more – please taste test)
1/4 cup fresh lemon juice, plus the zest of 1 lemon
3 eggs whisked
3 tbs coconut oil
1 tsp vanilla extract

Instructions
Preheat oven to 350-degrees F
In a small bowl, mix all the wet ingredients together
In a medium bowl, combine all the dry ingredients
Now pour the wet ingredients into the dry ingredients bowl, and stir into a batter
Let batter set for a few minutes, then stir it again
Grease a muffin tin or use muffin liners and fill each well or cup about two-thirds full
Bake about 15-20 minutes, or until a toothpick inserted into a muffin comes out clean
Serve and enjoy!

278. Strawberry chia Cupcake

Ingredients
½ c + 2 tbsp (56g) coconut flour
1 tsp xanthan gum
¾ tsp baking powder
¾ tsp baking soda
¼ tsp low sodium salt
1 tbsp (13g) chia seeds
1 tbsp (5g) lemon zest (about one medium)
1 tbsp (14g) coconut oil or unsalted butter, melted
1 large egg, room temperature
1 tsp vanilla extract
¼ c (60g) plain nonfat Greek yogurt
¼ c (60mL) agave
3 tbsp (45mL) freshly squeezed lemon juice (about one medium-large)
½ c (120mL) unsweetened vanilla almond milk
2 scoops (84g) vanilla protein powder
1 c (140g) frozen unsweetened strawberries, thawed slightly and diced

Instructions
Preheat the oven to 350°F, and lightly coat 9 standard-sized muffin cups with nonstick cooking spray. Whisk together the coconut flour, xanthan gum, baking powder, baking soda, salt, chia seeds, and lemon zest in a medium bowl. In a separate bowl, whisk together the coconut oil or butter, egg, and vanilla. Stir in the Greek yogurt until no large lumps remain. Stir in the agave, lemon juice, and almond milk. Mix in the protein powder. Add in the coconut flour mixture, stirring until fully incorporated. Let the batter rest for 10 minutes. Gently fold in the diced strawberries
Divide the batter between the prepared muffin cups. Bake at 350°F for 25-28 minutes, or until a toothpick inserted into the center comes out clean. Cool in the pan for 10 minutes before carefully turning out onto a wire rack.

Notes: Any milk (cow, soy, cashew, etc.) may be used in place of the almond milk.

279. Triple Coconut Cupcakes

Ingredients
1 cup almond flour
3 tbsp coconut flour
1 cup shredded coconut
1½ tsp baking powder
¼ tsp low sodium salt
5 drops stevia liquid (May need a few more – please taste test)
4 eggs, separated
¼ cup coconut oil
1 tbsp vanilla extract

Instructions
Preheat the oven to 350F. Grease a muffin tin or line with muffin cups.
Combine almond flour, coconut flour, shredded coconut, salt and baking powder in a medium mixing bowl.
Mix the egg yolks, stevia, coconut oil and vanilla extract in a small mixing bowl. Add to the almond flour mixture and combine thoroughly.
Using a hand mixer, whip the egg whites until they form stiff peaks.
Stir the egg whites into the rest of the ingredients, spoon the batter into the muffin tin.
Bake for 25 minutes (or until the tops are nicely browned and a tester comes out clean.

280. Lemon-Coconut Muffins

Ingredients
1 1/4 cup almond flour
1 cup shredded unsweetened coconut
2 tbs coconut flour
1/2 tsp baking soda
1/2 tsp baking powder
1/4 tsp low sodium salt
5 drops stevia liquid (May need a few more – please taste test)
1/3 cup fresh lemon juice, plus the zest of 1 lemon
1/4 cup full-fat coconut milk
3 eggs, whisked
3 tbs coconut oil
1 tsp vanilla extract

Instructions
Preheat oven to 350º F
In a small bowl, mix all the wet ingredients together
In a medium bowl, combine all the dry ingredients
Now pour the wet ingredients into the dry ingredients bowl, and stir into a batter
Let batter set for a few minutes, then stir it again
Grease a muffin tin or use silicone muffin liners (paper liners not recommended) and fill each well or cup about two-thirds full
Bake about 18-23 minutes. Test for doneness > insert toothpick into muffin center; if it comes out clean they're done
Serve and enjoy!

281. Chocolate Banana Muffins

Ingredients
2 medium super ripe bananas (each banana was 185 grams with the peel and 143 grams without)
5 drops stevia liquid (May need a few more – please taste test)
2 teaspoon vanilla extract
2 eggs
1/4 cup (56 grams) refined coconut oil, melted
200 grams (~2 cups but please weigh!) blanched almond flour
3 tablespoons (27 grams) coconut flour
1/3 cup (42 grams) Dutch process cocoa powder
1 teaspoon baking soda
1/4 teaspoon low sodium salt
1 cup (180 grams) semi-sweet chocolate chips ,additional mini chocolate chips for sprinkling, if desired

Directions
Preheat the oven to 350°F (175°C) and line a muffin tin with 12 muffin liners.
In a large bowl, mash the bananas with the bottom of a glass. They should almost be like a puree.
Add the stevia and vanilla and stir.
Add in the eggs and oil and stir until well combined.
In a medium bowl, mix together the almond flour, coconut flour, cocoa powder, baking soda and salt.
Stir just until combined and then stir in the chocolate chips.
Spoon the batter into the muffin liners and sprinkle on additional chocolate chips, if desired.
Bake for 18 minutes or until a toothpick inserted in the center comes out clean. Be careful not to confuse a melted chocolate chip with the batter.
Let the muffins cool for 5 minutes in the pan and then turn out onto a wire rack to cool completely.
Place in an airtight container and store in the refrigerator for up to 5 days.
Notes
Use can use unrefined coconut oil if you don't mind a slight coconut taste.

282. Delicious English Cupcakes

Ingredients
For the regular option
¼ cup almond or cashew flour
1 tablespoon coconut flour
¼ teaspoon baking soda
⅛ teaspoon low sodium salt
1 egg
½ tablespoon coconut oil
2 tablespoons water
For the cinnamon raisin option add the following to the regular option above
¼ teaspoon cinnamon
½ 5 drops stevia liquid (May need a few more – please taste test)
1½ tablespoons golden raisins

Instructions
Whisk together the dry ingredients in a small bowl.
Add the remaining wet ingredients and whisk again until fully incorporated.
Transfer the mixture into a greased microwave safe ramekin
Microwave for 2 minutes.
Remove from the ramekin, slice the muffin in half and toast for 2-3 minutes in a toaster oven.
Serve with softened butter.

283. Amazing Almond Flour Cupcakes

Ingredients:
2-1/2 cups almond flour or almond meal
¾ tsp baking soda
½ tsp low sodium salt
3 large eggs
⅓ cup unsweetened pumpkin puree, thawed winter squash puree, butternut squash puree, unsweetened apple sauce, or mashed very ripe banana
2 drops stevia, agave nectar or stevia
2 tablespoons coconut oil (melted) or vegetable oil
1 teaspoon vinegar (white or cider)
Optional Flavorings: 1 teaspoon extract (e.g., vanilla, almond), citrus zest, dried herbs (e.g., basil, dill), or spice (e.g., cinnamon, cumin)
Optional Stir-Ins: 1 cup fresh fruit (e.g., blueberries, diced apple) or ½ cup dried fruit/cacao nibs/chopped nuts/seeds or

Instructions:
Preheat oven to 350F. Line 10 cups in a standard 12-cup muffin tin with paper or foil liners.
In a large bowl whisk the almond flour, baking soda and salt (whisk in any dried spices or herbs at this point, if using).
In a small bowl, whisk the eggs, pumpkin, stevia, oil and vinegar (add any extracts or zest at this point, if using).
Add the wet ingredients to the dry ingredients, stirring until blended. Fold in any optional stir-ins, if using.
Divide batter evenly among prepared cups.
Bake in preheated oven for 14 to 18 minutes until set at the centers and golden brown at the edges.
Move the tin to a cooling rack and let muffins cool in the tin 30 minutes. Remove muffins from tin.

284. Delightful Cinnamon Apple Muffins

Ingredients:
1 cup unsweetened applesauce
4 eggs
1/4 cup coconut oil, melted
1 tsp vanilla
Stevia to taste
1/2 cup coconut flour
2 tsp cinnamon
1 tsp baking powder
1 tsp baking soda
1/4 tsp low sodium salt

Instructions:

Preheat oven to 350 degrees F. Line a muffin tin with liners. In a large bowl, add applesauce, eggs, coconut oil, stevia, and vanilla. Stir to combine.

Stir in the coconut flour, cinnamon, baking powder, baking soda, and low sodium salt. Distribute the batter evenly into the lined muffin tins, filling each about two-thirds of the way full.

Bake for 15-20 minutes, until a toothpick inserted into the center comes out clean. Serve warm or store in the refrigerator in a resealable bag.

285. Delish Banana Nut Muffins

Ingredients:
4 bananas, mashed with a fork (the more ripe, the better)
4 eggs
1/2 cup almond butter
2 tbsp coconut oil, melted
1 tsp vanilla
1/2 cup coconut flour
2 tsp cinnamon
1/2 tsp nutmeg
1 tsp baking powder
1 tsp baking soda
1/4 tsp low sodium salt

Instructions:
Preheat oven to 350 degrees F. Line a muffin tin with cups. In a large bowl, add bananas, eggs, almond butter, coconut oil, and vanilla. Using a hand blender, blend to combine.

Add in the coconut flour, cinnamon, nutmeg, baking powder, baking soda, and low sodium salt. Blend into the wet mixture, scraping down the sides with a spatula. Distribute the batter evenly into the lined muffin tins, filling each about two-thirds of the way full.

Bake for 20-25 minutes, until a toothpick comes out clean. Serve warm or store in the refrigerator in a resealable bag.

286. Apple Cinnamon Muffins

Ingredients
5 eggs
1 cup homemade applesauce (store bought should work too)
½ cup coconut flour
2-3 TBSP cinnamon
1 tsp baking soda
1 tsp vanilla (optional)
¼ cup coconut oil
5 drops stevia liquid (May need a few more – please taste test)

Instructions
Preheat the oven to 400 degrees F.
Grease a muffin pan with coconut oil.
Put all ingredients into a medium sized bowl and mix with immersion blender or whisk until well mixed.
Let sit 5 minutes.
Use ⅓ cup measure to spoon into muffin tins.
Bake 12-15 minutes until starting to brown and not soft when lightly touched on the top.
Let cool 2 minutes, drizzle with honey (if desired) and serve.

287. Apple Cardamom Cupcakes

Ingredients
½ cup applesauce
⅓ cup honey
4 large eggs
¼ cup coconut flour
½ teaspoon baking soda
¼ teaspoon salt
1 teaspoon cinnamon
¼ teaspoon nutmeg
¼ teaspoon cloves
½ teaspoon cardamom
For frosting:
1 cup coconut milk
1 cup honey
pinch of salt
1 teaspoon vanilla
2 tablespoons arrowroot powder
1 tablespoon water
1 cup coconut oil, melted
Instructions
Preheat oven to 350 degrees. Prepare muffin/cupcake pan with liners.
Using an electric mixer or by hand, combine applesauce, honey, and eggs until smooth.
Sift together all dry ingredients, making sure to get out any lumps in the coconut flour.
Combine dry and wet ingredients, mixing thoroughly.
Divide batter amongst 10-12 cupcake liners, filling each one about ⅔ of the way up.
Place in oven and bake for 35-45 minutes, or until top is lightly browned and toothpick comes out clean.
Meanwhile, begin making frosting. In a medium saucepan, heat coconut milk, honey, salt, and vanilla and allow to simmer for 10 minutes.
In a small bowl or ramekin, combine arrowroot powder and water to form a thick paste.
Add arrowroot mixture to pan, whisk vigorously, and bring to a boil.
Remove pan from heat and very slowly add melted coconut oil while mixing with an electric hand blender.
Allow pan to cool slightly, then place whole thing in refrigerator for at least an hour or until it is cool and has turned white.
Remove from refrigerator and use electric hand blender to whip until fluffy.
Spread a dollop on each cupcakes (this frosting is quite sweet, so you don't need a lot but let your tastes be the guide!).
Sprinkle with cinnamon for garnish.

Paleo Diet Recipes 365 Days Of Anti-Inflammatory Recipes
By Mercedes Del Rey

288. Chocolate Olive Oil Cupcakes

Ingredients
2 tablespoons cocoa powder
2 tablespoons coconut flour
1 teaspoon baking powder
1/4 teaspoon ground cinnamon
2 eggs
3 tablespoons honey
1/2 teaspoon vanilla extract
2 tablespoons olive oil
Icing
1 tablespoon coconut oil (melted)
1 tablespoon cocoa powder
1 tablespoon honey
Instructions for Cake
Preheat oven to 160 C.
Combine the cocoa, coconut flour, baking powder and cinnamon.
Add the eggs, honey, vanilla and olive oil.
Mix until smooth and well combined.
Spoon 4 lined cup cake tins.
Bake cupcakes for about 20 – 25 minutes.
Remove from the oven and allow to cool.
Instructions for Icing
Melt the coconut oil.
Mix in the cocoa powder.
Mix in the honey until all well combined.
Allow to harder then spread over muffins.
(Note: I didn't wait long enough for the icing to harder and the cupcake drank it up but it still tasted great!)

758 Pretty Vanilla Cup Cake

Ingredients
For the cupcakes:
¾ cup coconut flour
6 large eggs
¾ cup raw honey
½ cup melted coconut oil
1 tablespoon pure vanilla extract
¾ tsp baking powder
¼ tsp salt
For the icing:
1 can coconut milk (full fat) refrigerated overnight, scoop out coconut cream

1 tsp pure vanilla extract
2 heaping tablespoons pure coconut palm sugar or cane sugar

Instructions

Preheat the oven to 350 degrees.

Using a muffin pan, line each cup with a cupcake liner and spray generously with olive oil cooking spray or if not using cupcake liners grease very well with melted coconut oil.

In a bowl add the dry cupcake ingredients and mix to combine. In another small bowl whisk together the wet cupcake ingredients and add to the dry. Mix until completely smooth.

Pour the batter equally among the greased cups and bake in the oven for 16-18 minutes.

Allow the cupcakes to cook completely before removing from tin or removing from liners.

While the cupcakes are baking add the coconut cream to a large bowl with the vanilla and sugar. Use an electric beater and whip until frothy. Place in the fridge to chill.

Wait until the cupcakes are completely cooled and then pipe the coconut cream on each cupcake.

Place cupcakes back in the fridge for 3-4 hours to chill and the icing will firm up.

Top each cupcake with a halved fig slice, sprinkles, or other garnish of choice.

289. One-Bowl Coconut Flour Cupcakes

Ingredients
½ cup coconut flour
½ teaspoon baking powder
¼ teaspoon fine sea salt
4 large eggs (preferably brought to room temperature)
½ cup maple syrup, honey or agave nectar
⅓ cup coconut oil, warmed until melted (or vegetable oil of choice)
2 tablespoons dairy or nondairy milk of choice milk
2 teaspoons vanilla extract vanilla extract

Instructions
Preheat oven to 350°F.
IMPORTANT: Line 8 muffin cups with paper or silicone liners; spray insides of cups with nonstick cooking spray or oil/grease (to prevent sticking).
In a large bowl, whisk the flour, baking powder, and salt until blended. Whisk in the eggs, syrup, oil, milk, and vanilla until completely blended and smooth.
Divide the batter equally among the prepared muffin cups.
Bake in preheated oven for 18 to 22 minutes or until golden and a toothpick inserted in the center comes out clean.
Transfer baking tin to wire rack and cool 10 minutes.
Carefully remove the cupcakes from the tin and place on wire rack; cool completely.

Notes
Sore in an airtight container at room temperature for up to 2 days, in an airtight container in the refrigerator for up to 1 week, or freeze (unfrosted) for up to 2 months.

290. Meatloaf Cupcakes

Ingredients
1.5-2 pounds of ground beef (grass-fed if possible)
3 eggs
¼ cup almond flour (or enough to thicken- this will depend partially on the fat content of the meat and the texture of the almond flour)
1 teaspoon dried basil
1 teaspoon garlic powder
1 medium onion
2 tablespoons Worcestershire sauce
Salt and pepper to taste
5-6 sweet potatoes
¼ cup butter or coconut oil
1 teaspoon sea salt or Himalayan Salt

Instructions
Preheat the oven to 375 degrees
Finely dice the onion or puree in a blender or food processor.
In a large bowl, combine the meat, eggs, flour, basil, garlic powder, pureed onion, Worcestershire sauce, and salt and pepper and mix by hand until incorporated.
Grease a muffin tin with coconut oil or butter and evenly divide the mixture into the muffin tins to make 2-3 meat "muffins" per person. If you don't have a muffin tin, you can just press the mixture into the bottom of an 8x8 or 9x13 baking dish.
Put into oven on middle rack, and put a baking sheet with a rim under it, in case the oil from the meat happens to spill over (should only happen with fattier meats if at all)
For sweet potatoes: if they are small enough, you can put them into the oven at the same time, if not you can peel, cube and boil them until soft.
When meat is almost done, make sure sweet potatoes are cooked by whichever method you prefer, and drain the water if you boiled them.
Mix with butter and salt or pepper if desired and mash by hand or with an immersion blender.
Remove meat "muffins" from the oven when they are cooked through and remove from tin. Top each with a dollop of the mashed sweet potatoes to make it look like a cupcake.

291. Gluten Free Banana Nut Bread

Ingredients:
3 bananas, mashed, or 1 cup
3 eggs
1/2 cup almond butter
1/4 cup coconut oil, melted
1 tsp vanilla extract
1/2 cup almond flour
1/2 cup coconut flour
2 tsp cinnamon
1 tsp baking soda
1/4 tsp low sodium salt
1/2 cup chopped walnuts

Instructions:

Preheat the oven to 350 degrees F. Line a loaf pan with parchment paper. In a large bowl, add the mashed bananas, eggs, almond butter, coconut oil, and vanilla. Use a hand blender to combine.

In a separate bowl, mix together the almond flour, coconut flour, cinnamon, baking soda, and low sodium salt. Blend the dry ingredients into the wet mixture, scraping down the sides with a spatula. Fold in the walnuts.

Pour the batter into the loaf pan in an even layer. Bake for 50-60 minutes, until a toothpick inserted into the center comes out clean. Place the bread on a cooling rack and allow to cool before slicing.

292. Pumpkin crepes

ingredients
Apple Butter:
apples - 5 lb, peeled and sliced
cinnamon - to taste
Crepes:
egg yolk - 1
egg whites - 4
pure pumpkin puree - 1/3 cup
canned full-fat coconut milk - 1/3 cup
coconut flour - 3-4 tablespoons
arrowroot starch - 1/4 cup
pure vanilla extract - 1 teaspoon
ground allspice - 1/4 teaspoon
pure maple syrup - 3 tablespoons
instructions
Preheat oven to 425 degrees Fahrenheit.
Combine the apples and cinnamon to taste on 2 9 inch by 13 inch baking dishes.
Roast for 1-2 hours, stirring every 15 minutes, or until the apples have lost quite a bit of moisture.
Puree until smooth, adding water if necessary.
Preheat a nonstick skillet to 350 degrees Fahrenheit. Whisk together all crepe ingredients in a large bowl until smooth.
Lightly grease the skillet with coconut oil and add 4-5 tablespoons of batter, spreading it around with the back of a spoon.
Cook until the batter looks dry. Flip and cook until golden. Repeat with remaining batter.
Serve crepes with apple butter.

293. Red Coconut Smoothie

INGREDIENTS
1 cup coconut milk
1 frozen banana, sliced
2 cups frozen strawberries
1 teaspoon vanilla extract

INSTRUCTIONS
Add all ingredients to Blendtec and blend until smooth.

294. Briana's House Low Carb Chocolate Chip Cookies

INGREDIENTS
½ cup Briana's Baking Mix
½ cup oat fiber (use gluten free if necessary)
1 T THM Super Sweet Blend (or more to taste)
1 tsp. xanthan gum
½ tsp. baking soda
½ tsp. salt
8 T salted butter
4 T refined coconut oil
2 oz. cream cheese (full fat or reduced fat)
2 eggs
1 tsp. molasses
½ tsp. vanilla extract
¼ cup water
2 T heavy whipping cream
½ cup sugar free chocolate chips (such as Lily's brand) or chopped 85% dark chocolate

INSTRUCTIONS
Whisk the dry ingredients together.
Soften the butter, coconut oil, and cream cheese together, then beat them with the eggs, molasses, and vanilla until smooth. Add the water and whipping cream and beat again.
Add the dry ingredients to the wet ingredients and mix well. Stir in the chocolate chips by hand. Drop the dough by rounded tablespoons onto a cookie sheet, then smooth each cookie out thinly with the back of a spoon (each will be about 4 inches in diameter). Bake each pan of cookies at 375 degrees F for 7 minutes, then remove the pan from the oven and leave the cookies on it for 2 more minutes before transferring them to wire racks to cool completely. Store in the refrigerator. Yields 2 dozen cookies.
NOTES
Do not put cookie batter onto hot cookie sheets as you won't be able to spread the cookies out as well. Adjust the baking time according to how you like your cookies. This time is what worked best for me.

295. Coconut Vanilla Surprise

INGREDIENTS
1½ cups unflavored soy milk
2 tbsp. matcha green tea powder
stevia to taste
½ tsp. vanilla extract
¼ cup coconut milk
few dashes nutmeg

INSTRUCTIONS

Whisk together soy milk, matcha, sweetener and vanilla. Heat to desired temperate in a small saucepan on stove top or microwave in a microwave safe container.
Divide into mugs and froth.
Add coconut milk, and sprinkle with nutmeg. Serve.

296. Tempting Coconut Berry Smoothie

Ingredients:
½ Cup Frozen Blackberries
½ Frozen Banana
1 Teaspoon Chia Seeds
¼ Inch Piece Of Fresh Ginger
½ Cup Almond Coconut Milk
1 scoop of HEMP protein
2 Tablespoons Toasted Coconut

Instructions:
Combine all the ingredients in a blender and process until smooth.

297. Pineapple Coconut Deluxe Smoothie

Ingredients:
1 C pineapple chunks
1 C coconut milk
1/2 C pineapple juice
1 ripe banana
1/2 – 3/4 C ice cubes
Pure liquid stevia to taste
1 tablespoon hemp protein powder

Instructions:
In a blender, combine the pineapple chunks, coconut milk, banana, ice and pure liquid stevia.
Puree until smooth.
Pour into 2 large glasses.
Garnish with a pineapple wedge if desired.

298. Sumptuous Strawberry Coconut Smoothie

Ingredients:
1 cup coconut milk
1 frozen banana, sliced
2 cups frozen strawberries
1 teaspoon vanilla extract
1 tablespoon hemp protein powder

Instructions:
Add all ingredients to blender and blend until smooth.

299. Divine Peach Coconut Smoothie

Ingredients:
1 cup full fat coconut milk, chilled
1 cup ice
2 large fresh peaches, peeled and cut into chunks
Fresh lemon zest, to taste
1 tablespoon hemp protein powder

Instructions:
Add coconut milk, ice and peaches blender. Using a zester, add a few gratings of fresh lemon zest. Blend on high speed until smooth.

300. Raspberry Coconut Smoothie

Ingredients:
½ - 1 cup coconut milk (depending on how thick you like it)
1 medium banana, peeled sliced and frozen
2 teaspoons coconut extract (optional)
1 cup frozen raspberries
1 tablespoon hemp protein powder

optional: shredded coconut flakes, and stevia to taste

Instructions:
Add coconut milk, frozen banana slices and coconut extract to your blender.
Pulse 1-2 minutes until smooth.
Add frozen raspberries and continue to pulse until smooth.
Pour into your serving glass, top with a couple of raspberries and a little shredded coconut, and enjoy!

301. Sweet Melon

Ingredients
1/2 honeydew melon, cut into chunks (about 4 cups, or 1 1/2 lbs)
1/2 cup light coconut milk
1-2 leaves fresh mint (plus more for garnish)
1/2-1 tsp. fresh lime juice (or to taste)
1 cup ice
Drizzle of honey or coconut nectar, to taste (optional, depending on how sweet your melon is)

Directions
Cut your melon in half, remove the seeds, and slice away the outer rind. Cut the melon into chunks, and add to your blender along with the coconut milk, mint, lime, and ice. Blend until smooth. Taste, and adjust sweetness with honey or coconut nectar. Serve with a garnish of mint, or fresh melon slices.

302. CINNAMON Coconut Surprise

Ingredients
1/2 Cup Coconut Milk
4 Large Egg Yolks
1 Medium Banana
1/4 Cup Ice
1/2 tsp Cinnamon
Directions
Throw all of the ingredients into your high-speed blender and blast for 30 to 60 seconds until well combined. Enjoy right away while still fresh, and give a little stir if separation occurs.

303. Low Carb Fried Zucchini

INGREDIENTS:
3 medium zucchini or yellow squash
2 eggs
1 tablespoon water
1/3 cup coconut flour
1/4 cup powdered Parmesan cheese
vegetable oil, for frying
ranch dressing, for serving

DIRECTIONS:
Heat a 1/4 inch of oil in the bottom of a large skillet over medium heat.
Wash and slice the zucchini into thin rounds, about 1/8-1/4 inch thick.
Beat together the egg and water in a shallow bowl.
Stir together the coconut flour and Parmesan in a second shallow bowl.
Coat the zucchini in the egg and then dredge in the coconut mixture to coat.
Add a single layer of zucchini to the hot oil, being careful not to crowd the pan. Fry for 1-2 minutes on each side, until golden brown. Repeat with remaining zucchini.
Drain on a paper towel lined plate. Sprinkle with salt, if desired.
Serve with ranch dressing for dipping.

304. Slow Cooker Paleo Mexican Breakfast Casserole

Ingredients
1 sweet potato, cubed or shredded
8 eggs, whisked
1/2 pound turkey bacon
1 yellow onion, chopped
1 red bell pepper, chopped
1 (8 ounce) package mushrooms, chopped (optional)
1/2 packet taco seasoning (or make your own if you're strict paleo!)
Guacamole, salsa and jalapeno to garnish

Instructions
Fry turkey bacon in a skillet until crispy. Remove and set aside. Crumble when cool enough to touch.
In the same skillet, cook the onions until they are soft.
Transfer the bacon, onions, sweet potato, bell pepper, mushrooms and eggs to the slow cooker. Stir to combine.
Sprinkle in your taco seasoning and stir again to dissolve.
Cook on LOW for 6-8 hours. Slice and serve with guacamole, salsa and jalapeno!

305. Paleo Pumpkin Pie Smoothie

Ingredients
1 frozen banana
2 tbsp pumpkin puree
½ cup unsweetened almond milk
½ tsp vanilla extract
1 tsp honey
1 tbsp hemp hearts
¼ tsp cinnamon
¼ tsp cloves
¼ tsp nutmeg

Instructions

Combine all ingredients in a blender and process until smooth. I find it's easier on the blender if I break the frozen banana into smaller chunks before processing.

Pour into a tall glass and enjoy with your favourite book, your favourite music, or both!

Notes
Calories: 220
Total Fat: 6.4g
Saturated Fat: 0.8g
Carbs: 38.0g
Fiber: 6.1g
Protein: 5.6g

306. Paleo Cookie Butter

Ingredients
For the Cookie Butter
½ cup (128 grams) favorite nut butter, almond, cashew or macadamia
½ cup (128 grams) roasted sunflower butter, such as SunButter®
½ cup (128 grams) raw organic coconut butter, such as Artisana®
¼ cup (60 grams) organic ghee (you could also use coconut oil)
4 tablespoons (84 grams) organic raw honey*
1½ tablespoons (20 grams) 100% pure cocoa butter, I use Callebaut®, melted
1½ tablespoons (10.5 grams) organic coconut flour, such as Tropical Traditions®
1 teaspoon (5 grams) unsulphured molasses, such as Brer Rabbit®
1 teaspoon (about 2 grams) pure vanilla extract, such as Nielsen-Massey®
½ to 1 teaspoon ground cinnamon, such as Penzey's® Cinnamon
¼ teaspoon ground allspice
¼ teaspoon freshly grated whole nutmeg
Generous pinch of fine sea salt
Coconut palm sugar or pure stevia extract powder, to taste

*Do not serve raw honey to children under the age of 1 year.

For the Optional Mix-Ins for "Cookie Dough Butter"
Chopped dark chocolate 70% cocoa or more
Gluten free semi-sweet chocolate chips, such as Trader Joe's®
Chopped walnuts or pecans, toasted or not
Unsweetened shredded coconut, toasted or not

Special Equipment
Mini Prep Food Processor
Mason jar with lid, helpful but not necessary
Rubber spatula
Preparation
Place nut butter and SunButter into work bowl of prep food processor.
In a small saucepan over medium-low heat, melt and brown the coconut butter and ghee until golden brown, stirring constantly, about 3 minutes for a lighter "blonde" browned coconut butter or 5 minutes for a darker, rich browned coconut butter the color of dark coffee and cream. (The mixture will bubble and foam. Keep stirring.) Remove immediately from heat to prevent overbrowning or burning; stir and allow to cool until still warm (not room temp, but no longer hot). Note: It is important to remove the pan immediately when coconut butter mixture is browned to desired doneness as the residual heat will continue to cook the mixture.
Add browned coconut butter mixture to nut butter and SunButter®; process until well combined and smooth scraping down sides of bowl as necessary between pulses. The mixture will be very thin at this

point. Do not worry. Add honey, melted cocoa butter, coconut flour, molasses, vanilla extract, spices and salt; process until well combined and smooth. Taste and, if desired, sweeten additionally with coconut palm sugar or pure stevia extract.

Remove work bowl from processor unit. With a rubber spatula, or the plastic spatula that came with your processor unit, scrape and pour mixture into a small to medium bowl. Cover bowl with plastic food wrap and place in refrigerator until thickened, about 1 hour. Stir halfway through chilling time for an even chill. Remove from the fridge and stir to loosen. Transfer to Mason® jar, if desired, or other covered container for storing. Before serving add and stir in favorite mix-ins as desired, about a few tablespoons each. Keep stored in an airtight container, such as a Mason® jar, in refrigerator.

Notes

Tip: This homemade cookie butter softens upon room temperature. If you wish for a thicker cookie butter, either keep it chilled or simply stir in an additional 1 tablespoon of coconut flour (or more to desired thickness).

307. Paleo-friendly Coconut Chocolate Coffee Cake

Ingredients
What you'll need:
(all ingredients are available at Whole Foods or Natural Grocers/health sections; my ordering recommendations listed)
two medium-sized glass bowls for mixing & one square glass baking dish (8"x8")
coconut oil for greasing baking dish
4 eggs
½ cup full-fat coconut milk
¼ cup coconut butter
½ cup brewed coffee or espresso, as strong as you like
¼ cup grade B maple syrup
1 tsp. vanilla extract
½ cup almond flour
½ cup + 1 Tbs coconut flour
½ tsp. baking soda
pinch of sea salt
1 cup dark chocolate chips
½ cup unsweetened coconut flakes

What to do
Preheat the oven to 350° F.
Combine the first 6 ingredients (eggs, coconut milk, coconut butter, coffee, maple syrup, and vanilla) in a bowl. Mix them together. I always use my favorite kitchen tool, my stick blender, to do the mixing.
In a separate bowl, combine the almond flour, coconut flour, baking soda, and salt. Stir.
Add the liquid, a little at a time, to the dry ingredients, mashing and stirring the mixture until smooth.
Then, add half the chocolate chips to the mixture and stir them in.
Pour/push the mixture into the greased baking dish, smoothing it out with a spatula.
Top with coconut flakes, then chocolate chips.
Bake for 35 minutes, then allow it to cool.

308. Grain Free Steamed Christmas Puddings – GAPS & Paleo Friendly

Ingredients
150g sultanas
80g dried sour cherries or dried unsweetened cranberries, plus extra for garnish
100g currants
30g activated or raw almonds, roughly chopped
200g kombucha or freshly squeezed orange juice
zest of 1 orange
40g blanched almond meal
20g coconut flour
1/4 tsp nutmeg
1/2 tsp mixed spice
1/4 tsp cinnamon
55g tallow or coconut oil
40g apple, peeled & cored
2 eggs
1/4 tsp fine salt
1/4 tsp bicarb soda

Instructions
Weigh dried fruit and almonds into the Thermomix bowl, and add kombucha or orange juice.
Cook 6 mins/80C/reverse/speed soft. Remove to a large bowl and set aside to cool.
Place orange zest into clean, dry Thermomix bowl and chop 20 sec/speed 10.
Add almond meal, coconut flour, spices, salt, soda, apple, eggs and tallow or coconut oil into Thermomix bowl and mix 5 sec/speed 5. Scrape down sides of bowl.
Add soaked fruit and nuts back to bowl and mix 10 sec/reverse/speed 3.
Scoop mixture into silicone cupcake cups or small ramekins and place into the Varoma dish and tray, with lid on. Cups/ramekins should be about 3/4 full.
Place 500g water into Thermomix bowl and place Varoma in position. Cook 25 mins/Varoma/speed 2.
Allow puddings to cool, covered, and store in fridge until needed.
Drizzle with Coconut Vanilla Custard, with a dried cranberry or sour cherry on top for decoration.
Notes
I use my Thermomix to make these puddings - if you don't have a Thermomix, chop by hand, cook fruit gently on stovetop, and mix in remaining ingredients. Steam in a steamer or use traditional Christmas pudding cooking method.

309. Paleo Antioxidant Berry Shake

Ingredients
1/2 cup coconut milk
1/4 cup cold water
1/2 frozen banana
1/2 cup frozen raspberries
1/2 cup frozen blueberries
1 tbsp chia seeds

Directions
In a large cup (if using an immersion blender) or a blender, combine ingredients and blend until smooth. Add more water if necessary to reach desired consistency. Serve immediately.

Notes
Servings: 1
Difficulty: Easy

310. Perfect Paleo Loaf

Makes 1 traditional loaf
Ingredients:
- 1/2 cup + 2 tbsp coconut flour, sifted
- 2 tbsp finely ground golden flaxseed
- 1 tsp baking soda
- 6 eggs, separated
- 4 tbsp coconut oil, melted
- 1/2 cup coconut milk
- 1 tsp apple cider vinegar or lemon juice
- Low sodium salt (to taste)

Instruction:
1. Preheat your oven to 375 degrees F. Line a loaf pan with a sheet of parchment paper on it, brush some butter on the remaining uncovered sides.
2. In a large mixing bowl, sift together all dry ingredients; make sure all lumps are smoothed out.
3. Separate eggs, adding the yolks to the flour mixture and set aside the whites to a medium mixing bowl.
4. Add the melted coconut oil, coconut milk, and apple cider vinegar/lemon juice to the flour, mixing thoroughly. Expect the mixture to be dene and dry.
5. Whip egg whites with hand mixer until stiff peaks begin to form.
6. Fold egg whites into batter.
7. Spoon bread batter into a greased loaf pan. Smooth out the top with a spatula so that bread will bake evenly.
8. Bake for 35-40 minutes, covering bread with foil the last 5-10 minutes of baking.
9. Allow bread to cool for 5-10 minutes before transferring the bread to a cooling rack.
10. Slice and serve. Store any remaining bread in the refrigerator for up to 4 days.

Tips
It is very important to sift the coconut flour to remove any lumps, as it is a very dense flour.
Golden flaxseed as it adds a nice color to the bread making it look like a "multi-grain."
Whipping the egg whites allows the bread to be more fluffy and "slice-able."
This bread is not sweet. Many bread recipes have added honey or sweeteners, but if you want it to be a bit sweet, you can add a few drops of stevia.

311. Raw Pineapple Coconut Vegan Cheesecake

Crust:
4 dates, soaked until very soft1 cup dried organic, unsweetened coconut
Place soften dates and coconut in food processor and process until well blended.Pat into the bottom of an oiled 7 1/2 inch spring form pan.
Filling:
2 1/2 cups young Thai coconut flesh (about 5 young coconuts)1/4 cup coconut water (from the coconuts)1/3 cup raw agave nectar or liquid sweetener of choice1 cup coconut oil, softened2 cups fresh pineapple chunks, separated
In high-speed blender, pureé the coconut flesh and coconut water together until smooth.Add the agave, coconut oil. You want this to be quite smooth so blend away until it is.Add 1 cup of the pineapple chunks. Blend until incorporated.Pulse the remaining pineapple chunks in the food processor until well chopped. Drain.Stir the pineapple into the coconut mixture, pour over crust and let set up in the refrigerator for 4 hours. Move to freezer and leave until firm.

312. Nutritious Paleo Tortillas

Ingredients
1/4 cup coconut flour (40 g)
1/4 teaspoon baking powder
8 egg whites (240 g or 1 cup)
1/2 cup water
A pinch of low sodium salt
coconut oil (as needed, for greasing the press or pan)

Instructions
1. In a bowl mix all ingredients. Set aside for five minutes. The batter takes about that long to hydrate and thicken.
*If necessary grease your tortilla press or pan with coconut oil.

Make the tortillas:
1. In a preheated electric tortilla press: Pour about a little less than 1/4 cup of batter onto the tortilla press. Quickly smooth out using a heat resistant spoon, and press the top of the press down to distribute the rest of the batter. Cook until the indicator on the press goes off.
2. In a pan over medium heat: Pour a little less than 1/4 cup of batter onto the pan. Quickly smooth out using a heat resistant spoon. Cook for 1 to 2 minutes or until the edges of the tortilla start to turn golden brown. Then flip and cook for an additional minute or two.
3. Transfer tortillas to a plate and cover with a paper towel to keep warm.
4. Serve with desired toppings and do your best to keep away from within hungry doggy mouths.

313. Perfect Paleo Bananacado Fudge Cupcakes

Ingredients
2 1/2 c. almond butter
1 1/4 c. stevia (or you can lower this to 3/4 c. and add an additional banana)
2 lg ripe bananas
3 medium avocados
3 eggs, beaten
3/4 c. cocoa powder
1 tbsp. vanilla
1 tsp baking soda
2 tsp baking powder

Instructions
In a large bowl, mix the almond butter and stevia.
In a blender or mixer, beat the eggs, banana, vanilla, cocoa powder and avocado to form a mousse-like consistency.
Add baking soda and baking powder.
Fold into the almond butter to make batter.
Pour into mini-cupcake tin (use the paper, it really makes a difference)
Bake at 350 for 15-18 minutes depending on size and desired consistency.

314. Paleo Sticky Date Pudding Cupcakes

Ingredients
For the muffins
Coconut Butter grease the muffin tray with
10 tbsp water
12 dates
1 ½ ripe banana, peeled and roughly chopped
2 ½ -3 tbsp coconut flour
1 tbsp vanilla extract or essence or 1 fresh vanilla bean, seeds scraped out
2 eggs
5 drops stevia liquid (May need a few more – please taste test)
½ tsp baking powder
For the sticky date ganache
5-6 dates, chopped
½ of orange, juice only
3 tbsp almond milk (coconut milk or water can also be used)
1 tsp vanilla extract or essence
2 drops stevia
Fresh raspberries or strawberries for garnish

Instructions
Preheat oven to 185°C (365 °F).
Grease muffin tins with the butter and set aside.
Heat the dates and water in a small saucepan over low heat until the dates break down and thicken. Use a fork to mash them together and set aside.
Place the coconut flour, egg, banana, vanilla extract and baking powder in a blender or food processor and mix well until well combined and aerated.
Add the dates to the banana mixture and combine. Evenly distribute into the ramekins. Cook in the oven for about 20-22 minutes.
While the muffins are in the oven, place the sticky date ganache ingredients in a small saucepan over a low heat and cook for about 3-4 minutes or until the dates break down. Mash with a fork and whisk until thickened. Set aside.
Allow the muffins to rest for 5 minutes before removing them to a serving plate. Scoop a dollop of sticky date ganache paste on top and garnish with a few raspberries.

315. Vanilla Paleo Cupcakes

Ingredients:
Apple Cakes:
4 tablespoons (or ¼ cup) of Grass-Fed/Clarified Butter or Extra Virgin Coconut Oil
½ cup Unsweetened Applesauce
4 Eggs
1 teaspoon Vanilla Extract
5 drops stevia liquid (May need a few more – please taste test)
¾ cup Almond Flour
2 teaspoons Cinnamon
½ teaspoon Baking Powder
1/8 teaspoon low sodium Salt

Cinnamon Frosting:
1 cup room temperature coconut oil
5 drops stevia liquid (May need a few more – please taste test)
1 teaspoon Vanilla Extract
4 tablespoons (or ¼ cup) Arrowroot
2 teaspoons Coconut Flour
2 teaspoons Cinnamon
2 tablespoons Chilled Coconut Milk Cream

Topping:
½ Apple Thinly Sliced
Cinnamon for Dusting

Instructions
Apple Cakes:
Preheat oven to 350 degrees F. Line mini cupcake pan with 24 paper liners.
Melt the butter then whisk in with the applesauce, eggs, vanilla, and stevia.
Add the almond flour, cinnamon, baking powder, and salt to the wet ingredients and mix until evenly combined.
Evenly distribute into the 24 mini cupcake liners {about 1 tablespoon of batter each} and bake at 350 F for 18 – 19 minutes. The cakes are done when a toothpick can be poked in and come out without any batter on the stick.
Let the cool completely.

Cinnamon Frosting:
Whisk the shortening, stevia, vanilla, arrowroot, coconut flour, and cinnamon together until smooth.
Add the chilled coconut milk cream and whisk again until smooth.

Use immediately. Either spoon the frosting into a gallon plastic bag or a pastry bag.

Gently frost each cupcake with your desired amount of frosting.

Store the rest of the frosting in the refrigerator. Let it come to room temperature before you use as frosting again.

Topping:

Top each cupcake with a thin slice of fresh green apple and dust with ground cinnamon.

If you don't enjoy the cupcakes immediately, store them in an airtight container in the refrigerator.

316. Paleo Vanilla Cupcakes

Serves: 6 cupcakes
Ingredients
¼ cup coconut flour
⅛ teaspoon celtic sea salt
⅛ teaspoon baking soda
3 large eggs
¼ cup room temperature coconut oil
5 drops stevia liquid (May need a few more – please taste test)
1 tablespoon vanilla extract
Instructions
In a food processor, combine coconut flour, salt and baking soda
Pulse in eggs, shortening, honey and vanilla
Line a cupcake pan with 6 paper liners and scoop ¼ cup into each
Bake at 350° for 20-24 minutes
Cool for 1 hour
Frost with Paleo Chocolate Frosting
Serve

317. Paleo Chocolate Cupcake with "Peanut Butter" Frosting

Ingredients
Cake Ingredients
1/4 cup coconut flour
3 large eggs
1/4 cup cup unsweetened cacao powder
1/3 cup raw honey
1/4 cup coconut oil
1/2 tsp baking soda
1 tsp vanilla
Pinch of salt
Frosting Ingredients
3/4 cup sunflower butter
3/4 cup Tropical Traditions Palm Shortening –or– 3/4 cup organic butter
1/3 cup raw honey
2 tsp vanilla
pinch salt
Instructions
Make your frosting first
Frosting Instructions
Using a stand mixer or hand mixer, combine sunflower butter and shortening on medium-high speed until fluffy. Takes about 3 minutes.
Add honey, vanilla and pinch of salt. Whip on high for another couple of minutes.
It should look like frosting, thick enough to spread on a cupcake.
Place in fridge while you bake your cupcakes
Cake Instructions
Combine dry ingredients together in a bowl: coconut flour, cacao powder, baking soda, salt
Whisk eggs in another small bowl and add melted coconut oil, honey and vanilla
Combine with dry ingredients and mix
Pour into muffin cups of your choice
Bake at 350° F for 15-18 min.
Makes about 6-8 cupcakes
Once cooled, frost those yummy cakes!
We sprinkled on a few mini dark chocolate chips just for fun :)
Frosting holds up well, but refrigerate if you don't eat them all right away.

318. Addictive & Healthy Paleo Nachos

Ingredients
2 medium tomatoes, diced and seeded
2 tbsp fresh cilantro, chopped
1-2 tbsp lime juice
2 cups guacamole
2 tbsp green onions, chopped
For the sweet potato chips
3 large sweet potatoes
3 tbsp melted coconut oil
1 tsp salt
For the meat
1 medium yellow onion, finely diced
1 tbsp coconut oil
1 green chili, diced
1 lb. ground beef
2 cloves garlic, minced
1 tsp smoked paprika
1/2 tsp ground cumin
1 tbsp tomato paste
12 oz. canned diced tomatoes
1 tsp salt
1/2 tsp pepper

Instructions

To make the sweet potato chips, preheat the oven to 375 degrees F. Peel the sweet potatoes and slice thinly, using either a mandolin or sharp knife. In a large bowl, toss them with coconut oil and salt. Place the chips in a single layer on a rimmed baking sheet covered with parchment paper. Bake in the oven for 10 minutes, then flip the chips over and bake for another 10 minutes. For the last ten minutes, watch the chips closely and pull off any chips that start to brown, until all of the chips are cooked.

While the potato chips are baking, start preparing the beef. Melt the coconut oil in a large skillet over medium heat. Add the onion and chili to the pan and sauté for 3-4 minutes until softened. Add the ground beef and cook for 4-5 minutes, stirring regularly. Add the garlic, diced tomatoes, tomato paste, and remaining spices and stir well to combine. Bring the mixture to a simmer and then turn the heat down to medium-low. Cook, covered, for 20-25 minutes, stirring regularly.

Stir the chopped tomatoes, lime juice, and cilantro into the beef mixture. Adjust salt and pepper to taste. Remove from heat.

To assemble the nachos, form a large circle with the sweet potato chips on a platter. Add the beef mixture into the middle of the circle, and then top with guacamole and green onions.

Notes
Servings: 4-6
Difficulty: Medium

Paleo Diet Recipes 365 Days Of Anti-Inflammatory Recipes
By Mercedes Del Rey

319. Homemade Paleo Tortilla Chips

Ingredients
1 cup almond flour
1 egg white
1/2 tsp salt
1/2 tsp chili powder
1/2 tsp garlic powder
1/2 tsp cumin
1/4 tsp onion powder
1/4 tsp paprika

Directions
Preheat the oven to 325 degrees F. In a large bowl, combine all of the ingredients together until they form an even dough.
Roll out the dough between two pieces of parchment paper, as thinly as possible. Remove the top layer of parchment paper. Cut the dough into desired shapes for chips.
Move the dough, with the parchment paper, onto a baking sheet. Bake for 11-13 minutes, until golden brown. Remove from the oven and let cool 5 minutes. Use a spatula to remove the chips from the paper. Serve with guacamole or salsa.

320. Paleo Chocolate Cookies (I Can't Get Enough of These)

Ingredients
2 tbsp and 2 tsp coconut oil
3 oz. unsweetened dark chocolate
1/4 cup honey
2 eggs
1 1/2 tsp vanilla extract
1/2 cup coconut flour
1/2 tsp cinnamon

Instructions

In a large microwave-safe bowl, melt the coconut oil and chocolate in the microwave, stirring intermittently. Let cool for 5 minutes.

Add the eggs, vanilla, and honey to the chocolate mixture. Stir well to make sure not to scramble the eggs. Add in the coconut flour and cinnamon and mix well. Place in the refrigerator for approximately 30 minutes, until slightly hardened.

Preheat oven to 350 degrees F. Roll out the dough between two pieces of parchment paper until 1/4-inch thick. Cut out shapes with a cookie cutter and carefully place on a parchment-lined baking sheet. Repeat this step for remaining dough.

Bake cookies for 12-15 minutes. Allow to cool before serving.

Notes
Servings: approximately 18 cookies
Difficulty: Medium

321. Easy Paleo Shepherd's Pie

For the top layer
1 large head cauliflower, cut into florets
2 tbsp ghee, melted
1 tsp spicy Paleo mustard
Salt and freshly ground black pepper, to taste
Fresh parsley, to garnish
For the bottom layer
1 tbsp coconut oil
1/2 large onion, diced
3 carrots, diced
2 celery stalks, diced
1 lb. lean ground beef
2 tbsp tomato paste
1 cup chicken broth
1 tsp dry mustard
1/4 tsp cinnamon
1/8 tsp ground clove
Salt and freshly ground black pepper, to taste
Instructions

Place a couple inches of water in a large pot. Once the water is boiling, place steamer insert and then cauliflower florets into the pot and cover. Steam for 12-14 minutes, until tender. Drain and return cauliflower to the pot.

Add the ghee, mustard, salt, and pepper to the cauliflower. Using an immersion blender or food processor, combine the ingredients until smooth. Set aside.

Meanwhile, heat the coconut oil in a large skillet over medium heat. Add the onion, celery, and carrots and sauté for 5 minutes. Add in the ground beef and cook until browned.

Stir the tomato paste, chicken broth, and remaining spices into the meat mixture. Season to taste with salt and pepper. Simmer until most of the liquid has evaporated, about 8 minutes, stirring occasionally.

Distribute the meat mixture evenly among four ramekins and spread the pureed cauliflower on top. Use a fork to create texture in the cauliflower and drizzle with olive oil. Place under the broiler for 5-7 minutes until the top turns golden. Sprinkle with fresh parsley and serve.

Notes
Servings: 4
Difficulty: Medium

322. Paleo Apple Pie Cupcakes with Cinnamon Frosting

Ingredients:
WET INGREDIENTS
- 5 Eggs, room temperature
- 1/2 cup applesauce (you can make your own or use a sugar-free pre-made brand)
- 1/2 cup raw honey, melted
- 1/3 cup coconut oil, melted

DRY INGREDIENTS
- 1 1/4 cup finely ground blanch almond flour
- 1/2 cup coconut flour
- 1/2 tsp. sea salt
- 1/2 tsp. baking powder

FROSTING INGREDIENTS:
- 1 cup coconut oil
- 3 Tbsp. raw honey
- 2 tsp. cinnamon
- Dash sea salt

Equipment:
- Muffin tin
- 12 baking cups
- 2 medium mixing bowls
Hand mixe
- For

Directions:
1. Preheat oven to 350F. Line muffin pan with baking cups.
2. Combine all wet ingredients in a medium sized mixing bowl. Beat on medium with a hand mixer for about 30 seconds.
3. Combine all dry ingredients in another medium sized bowl. Mix together with a fork to break apart any clumps.
4. Add the dry ingredients to the wet ingredients and beat for about 20 seconds. Make sure all ingredients are combined.
5. Fill each lined muffin tin about 3/4 of the way full. Bake for 25-30 minutes or until a toothpick comes out clean in the center.
6. Take the cupcakes out of the oven and set aside to cool completely. All the way cooled! But feel free to sneak one to nibble on while the rest cool off.
7. Once the cupcakes have cooled, make the frosting! Combine all of the ingredients into a medium mixing bowl and beat on medium speed for about 30 seconds until well combines. Ice those cupcakes and get to eating!

323. Paleo French Toast with Blueberry Syrup

Ingredients
1 loaf Paleo bread (I used this recipe for Paleo Bread)
1/2 cup almond milk
2 eggs
1/2 tbsp vanilla
1 tsp cinnamon
Instructions
In a large bowl, whisk together the coconut milk, eggs, vanilla and cinnamon.
Heat a griddle or non-stick skillet to medium-high. Coat pan with coconut oil. Dip a slice of bread into the batter mixture to coat both sides, letting any excess drip off. Place the bread onto the pan and cook each side until slightly browned. Repeat with remaining bread. Serve warm.
Notes
Servings: 4
Difficulty: Easy

324. The Best Paleo Brownies (Chocolaty Goodness)

Ingredients
1 cup paleo-friendly almond butter
1/3 cup maple syrup
1 egg
2 tbsp ghee
1 tsp vanilla
1/3 cup cocoa powder
1/2 tsp baking soda

Instructions
Preheat the oven to 325 degrees F. In a large bowl, whisk together the almond butter, syrup, egg, ghee, and vanilla. Stir in the cocoa powder and baking soda.

Pour the batter into a 9-inch baking pan. Bake for 20-23 minutes, until the brownie is done, but still soft in the middle.

Notes
Servings: 6
Difficulty: Easy

325. Paleo Chocolate Cranberry Muffins

INGREDIENTS
200 grams almond flour (about 2 cups)
⅓ cup cacao powder
2 tablespoons coconut sugar
½ teaspoon baking soda
⅛ teaspoon salt
3 eggs
¼ cup honey
¼ cup ghee, melted
1 teaspoon vanilla extract
1 teaspoon apple cider vinegar
½ cup cranberries, thawed if frozen

INSTRUCTIONS
Preheat oven to 325 degrees and grease or line muffin tin.
Combine almond flour, cacao, coconut sugar, baking soda, and salt in a large bowl. Combine eggs, honey, ghee, vanilla, and apple cider vinegar in medium bowl. Stir wet ingredients into dry ingredients, then fold in cranberries.
Using a large ice cream or cookie scoop, fill muffin cups ¾ full.
Bake 20 - 25 minutes, until toothpick inserted in center comes out clean.

326. Salt and Vinegar Zucchini Chips

Ingredients
4 cups thinly sliced zucchini (about 2-3 medium)
2 tablespoons extra virgin olive oil
2 tablespoons white balsamic vinegar
2 teaspoons coarse sea salt

Instructions
Use a mandolin or slice zucchini as thin as possible.
In a small bowl whisk olive oil and vinegar together.
Place zucchini in a large bowl and toss with oil and vinegar.
Add zucchini in even layers to dehydrator then sprinkle with coarse sea salt.
Depending on how thin you sliced the zucchini and on your dehydrator the drying time will vary, anywhere from 8-14 hours.
To make in the oven: Line a cookie sheet with parchment paper. Lay zucchini evenly. Bake at 200 degrees F for 2-3 hours. Rotate half way during cooking time.
Store chips in an airtight container.

327. Nutritious Paleo Tortillas

Ingredients
1/4 cup coconut flour (40 g)
1/4 teaspoon baking powder
8 egg whites (240 g or 1 cup)
1/2 cup water
A pinch of low sodium salt
coconut oil (as needed, for greasing the press or pan)

Instructions
1. In a bowl mix all ingredients. Set aside for five minutes. The batter takes about that long to hydrate and thicken.
*If necessary grease your tortilla press or pan with coconut oil.
Make the tortillas:
1. In a preheated electric tortilla press: Pour about a little less than 1/4 cup of batter onto the tortilla press. Quickly smooth out using a heat resistant spoon, and press the top of the press down to distribute the rest of the batter. Cook until the indicator on the press goes off.
2. In a pan over medium heat: Pour a little less than 1/4 cup of batter onto the pan. Quickly smooth out using a heat resistant spoon. Cook for 1 to 2 minutes or until the edges of the tortilla start to turn golden brown. Then flip and cook for an additional minute or two.
3. Transfer tortillas to a plate and cover with a paper towel to keep warm.
4. Serve with desired toppings and do your best to keep away from within hungry doggy mouths.

328. Perfect Paleo Bananacado Fudge Cupcakes

Ingredients
2 1/2 c. almond butter
1 1/4 c. stevia (or you can lower this to 3/4 c. and add an additional banana)
2 lg ripe bananas
3 medium avocados
3 eggs, beaten
3/4 c. cocoa powder
1 tbsp. vanilla
1 tsp baking soda
2 tsp baking powder

Instructions
In a large bowl, mix the almond butter and stevia.
In a blender or mixer, beat the eggs, banana, vanilla, cocoa powder and avocado to form a mousse-like consistency.
Add baking soda and baking powder.
Fold into the almond butter to make batter.
Pour into mini-cupcake tin (use the paper, it really makes a difference)
Bake at 350 for 15-18 minutes depending on size and desired consistency.

329. Incredibly Easy Paleo Chicken Soup

Ingredients
4 cups (946 mL) chicken broth
2 inch (5.1 cm) piece fresh ginger, sliced into thin coins
1 inch piece (2.5 cm) fresh turmeric*, sliced into thin coins
3 cloves garlic, peeled & smashed
½ teaspoon (3 mL) fish sauce
2 cups (280 g) cooked shredded chicken
4 ounces (113 g) shiitake mushrooms, sliced
3 green onions (48 g), white and light green parts, thinly sliced
1 medium carrot (40 g), julienned or shredded
Sea salt, to taste
Optional: 1 cup (227 g) zucchini noodles, kelp noodles, or mountain yam shiritaki noodles
Optional: Paleo Sriracha for drizzling
Instructions

Pour the chicken broth into a medium pot, and add the ginger, turmeric, garlic and fish sauce. Bring to a boil, then reduce to a simmer for 20 to 30 minutes to really infuse the broth with flavor. Note: If using turmeric powder (ground turmeric), start with ¼ teaspoon (0.5 gram), and increase to ½ teaspoon (1 gram), depending on your preference. I find turmeric powder to be insanely potent, much more so than the fresh root, so always add less and bump it up if you'd like. While the broth is simmering, prepare the rest of the ingredients.
Using a slotted spoon, remove the ginger, turmeric and garlic. Discard. Or, if you like to live dangerously, leave it all in the soup and pick around it while you're eating (like I did in the photo). Just be aware: Biting into a large chunk of ginger, turmeric or garlic is usually not pleasant.
Add the chicken, mushrooms, green onions, carrot and if desired, your noodles. Heat about 5 minutes on medium-low or until everything is warmed through. Taste and adjust the seasoning with sea salt.
Serve with a drizzle of sriracha for some extra heat.
Notes
*If you can't find fresh turmeric root, sub in ¼ teaspoon (0.5 g) turmeric powder. When working with any form of turmeric, take care because it stains hands, clothing and porous surfaces.

330. Paleo Chicken Soup

Ingredients:
2 pounds uncooked chicken breasts/thighs
1 pound diced carrots
2 medium sweet potatoes cubed (I love white sweet potatoes!) or 1 pound parsnips diced
6 ribs/stalks celery chopped
1 onion diced
2-3 garlic cloves diced finely
2 to 3 tsp sea salt
1/2 to 1 tsp black pepper
4 cups chopped kale or collards.
6 to 8 cups Chicken Broth/Stock
Optional: 1 to 2 tbsp dried herbs (rosemary, thyme, sage)

Directions:
Grab your slow cooker or giant stock pot. Add all of ingredients except for the broth.
If you like a thicker soup, add just enough broth to barely cover the ingredients. If you enjoy a more broth-y soup add the full amount of broth.
Slow Cooker: 7 to 8 hours on low, 3-4 hours on high. Stovetop: Bring the soup to a boil, cover, and reduce to simmer (low) – leave for one hour.
Once the soup is finished cooking (chicken is cooked through and veggies are soft) remove the chicken and shred or chop it.

331. Paleo Chicken Soup with Nuddles

Ingredients
2 tablespoons coconut oil
1 onion, minced
1 carrot, peeled and sliced thin
1 rib celery, sliced
2 teaspoons minced fresh thyme or 1/2 teaspoon dried
2 1/2 quarts homemade bone broth
3 cups shredded chicken
1/4 cup minced fresh parsley
3-4 eggs, lightly beaten
sea salt and pepper to taste

Instructions
1. Heat the oil in a large Dutch oven over medium-high heat until shimmering. Add the onion, carrot, and celery and cook until softened, 3-4 minutes. Stir in the thyme, bone broth, and chicken. Bring to a simmer and cook until the vegetables are tender, about 15 minutes. Stir in parsley.
2. Stir soup gently so that it is moving in a circle. Pour beaten eggs into soup in a slow steady stream. This will create "noodles" for the soup. Remove soup from heat and let stand for 2 minutes. Break up the eggs using a fork. Season with sea salt and pepper to taste before serving.

332. PALEO CROCK POT CHICKEN SOUP

Ingredients
1 medium onion, chopped
3 celery stalks, diced
3 carrots, diced
1 teaspoon apple cider vinegar
1 tablespoon herbes de Provence, or several sprigs fresh herbs
2 organic chicken breasts, bone-in, skin-on
2 organic chicken thighs, bone-in, skin-on
1 teaspoon sea salt
½ teaspoon fresh ground pepper
3-4 cups filtered water

Instructions
Layer all ingredients in crock pot in order listed, making sure chicken is bone side down on top of vegetables. Add enough water to cover vegetables and come half way up chicken, between 3 and 4 cups.
Cook on low for 6-8 hours.
Remove chicken and let cool slightly. Remove skin and bones. Shred chicken meat and add back to soup in crock pot. Adjust seasonings, reheat, and serve.

333. Paleo Stuffed Breakfast Peppers

Ingredients
2 bell peppers – your choice of colour
4 eggs
1 cup white mushrooms
1 cup broccoli
¼ tsp cayenne pepper
Salt and pepper, to taste
Directions
Preheat oven to 375 degrees Fahrenheit.
Dice up your vegetables of choice.
In a medium sized bowl, mix eggs, salt, pepper, cayenne pepper, and vegetables.
Cut peppers into equal halves. A tip: Try to buy peppers that are symmetrical and have somewhat flat sides – this makes it easier for them to balance while baking.
Core the peppers so that they're clean enough to add the filling.
Pour a quarter of the egg / vegetable mix into each pepper halve, adding more vegetables to the top to fill in any empty space.
Place on baking sheet and cook approximately 35 minutes or until eggs are cooked to your liking.
Serve and enjoy! I personally like mine with a dash of hot sauce on top.
Notes
This recipe makes 2 servings.
Nutrition Facts Per Serving
Calories: 186
Total Fat: 9.4g
Saturated Fat: 2.8g
Carbs: 12.1g
Fiber: 4.0g
Protein: 14.6g

334. Blushing Beet Salad

Ingredients:
2 large beets, washed and stems cut off
1 cup carrots, peeled and cooked
1 tbsp cilantro, chopped
1 tbsp diced onion
2 tbsp paleo mayonnaise
Low sodium salt and pepper

Instructions:
Boil beets in water until soft, about 50 minutes. Peel and cut into small 1/2" cubes. Cook carrots until tender and cut into bite size cubes. Combine diced onion, carrots, beets, mayonnaise, cilantro, low sodium salt and pepper.

335. Cheeky Chicken Salad

Ingredients:
olive oil spray
2 tsp olive oil
16 oz (2 large) skinless boneless chicken breasts, cut into 24 1-inch chunks
Low sodium salt and pepper to taste
4 cups shredded romaine
1 cup shredded red cabbage
For the Skinny Cheeky Sauce:
2 1/2 tbsp paleo mayonnaise
2 tbsp scallions, chopped fine plus more for topping
1 1/2 tsp chilli flakes

Instructions:
Preheat oven to 425°F. Spray a baking sheet with olive oil spray.

Season chicken with low sodium salt and pepper, olive oil and mix well so the olive oil evenly coats all of the chicken.

Meanwhile combine the sauce in a medium bowl. When the chicken is ready, drizzle it over the top and enjoy!!

336. Melting Mustard Chicken

Ingredients:
8 small chicken thighs, skin removed
3 tsp mustard powder
1 tbsp paleo mayonnaise
1 clove garlic, crushed
1 lime, squeezed, and lime zest
3/4 tsp pepper
Low sodium salt
dried parsley

Instructions:

Preheat oven to 400°. Rinse the chicken and remove the skin and all fat. Pat dry …place in a large bowl and season generously with low sodium salt. In a small bowl combine mustard, mayonnaise, lime juice, lime zest, garlic and pepper. Mix well. Pour over chicken, tossing well to coat.

Spray a large baking pan with a little Pam to prevent sticking since all the fat and skin was removed from chicken. Place chicken to fit in a single layer.

Top the chicken with dried parsley. Bake until cooked through, about 30-35 minutes.

Finish the chicken under the broiler until it is golden brown. Serve chicken with the pan juices drizzled over the top.

337. Easy Paleo Spaghetti Squash & Meatballs

Ingredients
One medium spaghetti squash.
One pound of ground Italian sausage.
One can of tomato sauce, I used a 14 ounce can.
2 tbsp of hot pepper relish (optional).
4 to 6 cloves of garlic, whole.
2 tbsp of olive oil.
Italian seasoning (Oregano, Basil, Thyme) to taste, I used about 2 tsp

Instruction
Make sure you use a large 6 quart slow cooker for this recipe.
Dump your tomato sauce, olive oil, garlic, hot pepper relish and Italian seasoning into your slow cooker and stir well.
Cut your squash in half and scoop out the seeds.
Place your 2 squash halves face down into your slow cooker.
Roll your ground sausage into meatballs, then fit as many as you can in the sauce around the squash. I was able to work in about a half pound worth.
Cook on High for 3 hours or cook on low for 5 hours.
Use a large fork to pull the "spaghetti" out of your squash, then top with your meatballs and sauce.
Garnish with parsley if you feel fancy, and enjoy!

338. Paleo Pulled Pork Sliders

Ingredients
1. Large pork roast
2. 1 large onion, sliced
3. 3 minced garlic cloves
4. 2 tsp cumin
5. 2 tsp chili powder
6. 1 tsp pepper
7. 2 tsp oregano
8. 1 tsp paprika
9. 1/2 tsp cayenne pepper
10. 1/2 tsp cinnamon
11. 2 tsp sea salt
12. juice of 1 lime
13. juice of 1 lemon

Instructions
1. Stir together the spices and rub all over the roast. Lay the onion slices down on the bottom of the slow cooker, and squeeze half of the fruit juices in. Put the roast in the crockpot and squeeze the remaining lime and lemon juice over it. Cook on low overnight or throughout the day about 8 hours (you really can't overcook it to be honest). When done, shred it with two forks until it's completely 'pulled'.

The "Buns"
1. 1 large sweet potato (try to go for a nice evenly round one, remember the diameter will be the size of your sliders)
2. 2 tbsp coconut oil
3. 1/4 tsp cumin
4. 1/4 tsp paprika
5. dash of sea salt

Instructions
1. Slice the sweet potato into 1/4" thick rounds. Lay them out on a parchment paper-lined cookie sheet.
2. Brush each slice with coconut oil and sprinkle with the spices, then flip and do the same on the other side.
3. Bake at 425 degrees Farenheit for 35 minutes until golden brown on the outside and cooked all the way through, flipping halfway through. You may need to crank it up to 450 if your oven isn't nice and sizzly.
4. Top a patty with pulled pork, and add any other toppings or sauces you'd like (I just used some lettuce from our garden).
5. Finish with the top patty and enjoy your delightful little sliders!

339. Basic Balsamic Steak Marinade

Ingredients
1 lb. flank steak
Salt and pepper
2 cloves garlic, minced
1/2 tbsp oregano
1/2 tbsp rosemary
1 tsp Paleo mustard
1/4 cup balsamic vinegar
1 tsp honey
1/2 cup extra virgin olive oil

Instructions

Stir together the garlic, oregano, rosemary, mustard, vinegar, honey, and olive oil.

Salt and pepper the steak and place in a shallow dish, then pour the marinade over the steak. Cover and place in the refrigerator for 3-12 hours.

To cook the steak, heat the grill to medium and cook each side approximately 4-5 minutes, or until desired doneness. Let stand for about 5 minutes before slicing and serving.

Notes
Servings: 3
Difficulty: Medium

340. Lemon Tilapia Ajillo

Ingredients:
6 (6 oz each) tilapia filets
4 cloves garlic, crushed
2 tbsp olive oil
2 tbsp fresh lemon juice
4 tsp fresh parsley
Low sodium salt and pepper
cooking spray
large romaine lettuce, 1 grated carrot, half grated onion, handful baby tomatoes
Basic Paleo Dressing:
2 tblspoon best quality olive oil
1 tbspn apple cider vinegar
Squirt of fresh lemon juice
Half teaspoon garlic powder and half teaspoon onion powder
Black pepper to taste
Instructions:
Preheat oven to 400°.
Melt butter on a low flame in a small sauce pan. Add garlic and saute on low for about 1 minute. Add the lemon juice and shut off flame.
Spray the bottom of a baking dish lightly with cooking spray. Place the fish on top and season with low sodium salt and pepper. Pour the lemon butter mixture on the fish and top with fresh parsley. Bake at 400° until cooked, about 15 minutes.
Serve with a mixed salad and paleo dressing

341. Paleo crock Bone Broth

Ingredients
2 bags beef bones or 2 chicken carcasses
1 large onion, sliced in half
1 head garlic, sliced in half
3-4 slices celery, cut into 1" pieces
1 cup baby carrots
1 large handful fresh thyme or sage
1 tablespoon apple cider vinegar per pound of bones
Water

Instructions
Place all ingredients in a 5-7 quart slow cooker. Fill with enough water to completely immerse. Cover and cook for 12 hours on low.
Remove large bones with tongs, and pour the broth through a slotted spoon into freezer-safe containers or mason jars. Cool and freeze what you don't plan to use within 4 days. Frozen bone broth will last up to 6 months in the freezer. Enjoy!

342. Paleo Phobroth

Ingredients
1. 1 onion, halved
2. 2" fresh ginger, halved lengthwise
3. 1 teaspoon avocado oil
4. 6 cups of Bare Bones Beef Broth
5. 4 cups of filtered water
6. 2 tablespoons fish sauce
7. 1 teaspoon sea salt

Spices
1. 1 cinnamon stick
2. 6 whole star anise
3. 5 whole cloves
4. 2 cardamom pods
5. 1 tablespoon fennel seeds

Directions:
Wrap the above ingredients in cheesecloth and securely tie
1. 1.5 lbs. of sirloin, very thinly sliced
2. 3 to 4 large parsnips, peeled

Toppings
1. lime wedges
2. chilli peppers
3. basil
4. mint
5. cilantro
6. bean sprouts
7. hot sauce

coconut aminos

Char your ginger and onions, by placing them on a baking sheet in the highest position of your oven (toaster oven works great for this!). Turn your broiler on high. Brush the onions and ginger with avocado oil and place them on your baking sheet. Broil for 10 minutes and then turn and continue to broil for another 5 to 10 minutes.

In a large pot, add the broth, filtered water, the charred onions and ginger, fish sauce, salt and spices wrapped in cheesecloth. Cover the broth and bring to a light boil and then turn down to a simmer. Continue simmering for 1 to 1.5 hours.

Towards the end of your broth's cooking time, slice the parsnips and thinly slice the meat and set in the fridge, until ready to use.

Put the broth through a mesh strainer to remove the ginger, onions and spices. Return it to the pot. Taste the broth and adjust the seasoning. The broth is the star of the show, so make sure it tastes great. You can add more salt or fish sauce, if it is not salty enough. If it is too salty, you can even add a little bit of honey to balance it out.

Bring your broth back to a light boil. Add the sliced meat to the strained broth and allow it to cook through. This is how I do it. Some people place the meat in individual bowls and pour the piping hot broth over it. Which I think is the more traditional method, but I prefer to cook it all in the large pot. Add parsnips to the bottom of each bowl, ladle hot piping broth and meat into each bowl. Garnish with your favourite toppings and enjoy!

343. Fantastic Paleo Broth

Ingredients
1 quart beef bone broth (see above notes)
1 piece ginger root
1 onion
1 beef steak thickly cut
2 whole star anise
1 tsp. fennel
1 tsp. coriander
2 whole cloves
1 stick cinnamon
1 cardamom pod
2 Tbsp. fish sauce I used the liquid that comes off from my homemade anchovies.
Garnishes spicy peppers, lime slices, sprouts, basil leaves, etc.

Instructions
Begin by making your beef bone broth as explained above. You can either add in your spices during that process or separate out some broth and continue with the recipe as follows.
Simmer your broth in a pot on the stove with your spice blend added in. I usually put my spices into a cotton bag to make for easier straining later on. As you simmer the broth, skim off any foam that comes to the top.
Meanwhile, wash both your ginger root and your (peeled) onion, slice them in half, and place them on a baking sheet in your oven.
Broil them until they get dark on top.
Once your ginger and onion are ready, add them to your simmering broth to give it more flavour.
Keep simmering for around half an hour, or until the soup has absorbed the flavours of the spices to your liking. At this point, I like to add in the fish sauce to taste. I start by adding one tablespoon and then taste it and then add more, a little bit at a time, if I think it needs it.
Remove your broth from the stove and remove the ginger and onion. I like reserving the onion for adding back to the soup later on. Strain the broth if necessary to get out any of the remaining spices, and put the broth back into the pot.
Meanwhile, I like to sear the outside of the beef that I will be adding to the pho. Many people like to thinly slice it raw and add it to the soup that way. I prefer to sear the edges first, leaving it very rare inside.
When you are ready to serve the soup, add the broth to each bowl. Thinly slice the seared beef and place the thin slices on top of the soup. The heat of the soup will help lightly cook the thin slices.
Serve with garnishes that each person can add to their bowl of soup as desired.

344. Tasty Tomato Tilapia

Ingredients:
2 tbsp extra virgin olive oil
4 (6 oz) tilapia filets
2 garlic cloves, crushed
2 shallots, minced
2 tomatoes, chopped
2 tbsp capers
1/4 cup white wine
Low sodium salt and fresh pepper

Instructions:
Brush fish with 1 tbsp olive and season with low sodium salt and pepper.
In a medium sauté pan, heat remaining olive oil. Add garlic and shallots and sauté on medium-low about 4-5 minutes. Add tomatoes and season with low sodium salt and pepper. Add wine and sauté until wine reduces, about 5 minutes. Add capers and sauté an additional minute.
Meanwhile, set broiler to low and place fish about 8 inches from the flame. Broil until fish is cooked through, about 7 minutes.
Place fish on a platter and top with tomato caper sauce.
Eat with a green salad and paleo dressing

345. Beet Sprout Divine Salad

Ingredients:
1/2 pound Brussels sprouts, ends trimmed, outer leaves removed, and cut in half lengthwise
4 small red beets, tops trimmed to 1/2-inch, washed and cut in half lengthwise
4 tablespoons plus 1/3 cup extra virgin olive oil
1 tablespoon paleo Dijon mustard
Stevia to taste
Squeeze of lemon juice
Coarse low sodium salt
Grinding coarse black pepper
1 small red onion thinly sliced into rings

Instructions:
Preheat the oven to 350.
Pour 2 tablespoons olive oil in a baking dish. Toss the Brussels sprouts in the oil; sprinkle them with low sodium salt and pepper and roast them for 20 minutes.
Turn them once during the cooking. They are done when a small knife easily pierces them.
Pour 2 tablespoons of the olive oil on a sheet of aluminum foil and place
it on a baking sheet. Toss the beet halves in the olive oil. Sprinkle them with low sodium salt and pepper and, keeping them in a single layer, fold and seal the foil over them. Bake on the baking sheet until a knife easily pierces them.
When cool enough to handle, peel the beets and cut them into 1/4-inch slices.
Meanwhile combine the 1/3 cup olive oil, mustard, stevia, lemon juice and low sodium salt and pepper in a small bowl.
Toss the Ingredients, add the dressing and serve at room temperature.

346. Paleo Keto Bone Broth

Ingredients
3.3 lb oxtail (1.5 kg) or mixed with assorted bones (chicken feet, marrow bones, etc.)
2 medium carrots
1 medium parsnip or parsley root
2 medium celery stalks
1 medium white onion, skin on
5 cloves garlic, peeled
2 tbsp apple cider vinegar or fresh lemon juice
2-3 bay leaves
1 tbsp salt (I like pink Himalayan)
8-10 cups water, enough to cover the bones, no more than 2/3 capacity of your pressure cooker or 3/4 capacity of your Dutch oven or 3/4 capacity of your slow cooker

Instructions
Peel the root vegetables and cut them into thirds. Halve the onion and peel and halve the garlic cloves. Keeping the onion skin on will help the broth get a nice golden colour. Cut the celery into thirds. Place everything into the pressure cooker (or slow cooker) and add the bay leaves.
Add the oxtail and bones. You can use any bones you like: chicken, pork or beef, with or without meat. Because I used chicken and turkey bones with some skin on, the fat ended up being quite runny. You can still use it for cooking but I binned it.
Oxtail is rich in gelatin and contains more fat. Although traditional bone broth is made just from bones, especially beef marrowbones, I found oxtail to give the best flavor to my broth. The advantage of using oxtail is that it will yield 3 superfoods: bone broth, tender oxtail meat and tallow. Tallow is great when used for cooking the same way as ghee or lard.
Add 8-10 cups of water or up to 2/3 of your pressure cooker, slow cooker or Dutch oven, vinegar or freshly squeezed lemon juice and bay leaves. Make sure you use the vinegar or lemon juice – this will help release more minerals into the broth.
Add pink Himalayan salt (whole or powdered). While adding vinegar to bone broth helps release the gelatin and minerals from the bones, pink Himalayan rock salt adds extra minerals, including potassium!
Pressure Cooker: Lock the lid of your pressure cooker and turn to high pressure / high heat. Once it reaches high pressure (either you have an indicator or in case of old pressure cookers, see a small amount of vapor escaping through the valve), turn to the lowest heat and set the timer for 90 minutes.
Dutch oven or Slow cooker: Cover with a lid and cook for at least 6 hours (high setting) or up to 10 hours (low setting). To release even more gelatine and minerals, you can cook it up to 48 hours. To do that, you'll have to remove the oxtail using thongs and shred the meat off using a fork. Then, you can place the bones back to the pot and cook up to 48 hours.
Pressure cooker: When done, take off heat and let the pressure release naturally for about 10-15 minutes. Remove the lid.

Remove the large bits and pour the broth through a strainer into a large dish. Discard the vegetables and set the meaty bones aside to cool down.

When the meaty bones are chilled, shred the meat off the bone with a fork. If there is any gelatine left on the bones, you can reuse the bones again for another batch of bone broth. Just keep in the freezer and add some new pieces when making bone broth again. Use the juicy oxtail meat in other recipes (on top of lettuce leaves, with cauli-rice or as omelet filling) or eat with some warm bone broth.

Use the broth immediately or place in the fridge overnight, where the broth will become jelly. Oxtail is high in fat and the greasy layer on top (tallow) will solidify. Simply scrape most of the tallow off (as much as you wish).

Keep the broth in the fridge if you are planning to use it over the next 5 days. For future uses, place in small containers and freeze.

347. Faux Paleo Napoleon

Ingredients:
Dough:
2 ½ cups almond flour
½ teaspoon baking soda
¼ teaspoon sea salt
½ cup + 2 tablespoons organic palm shortening, slightly melted so that it's easy to mix
2 tablespoons honey
1 tablespoon vanilla extract
Filling:
2 cups almond flour
½ cup organic palm shortening or butter (I used shortening. Can't vouch for the results if butter is used, but I don't see why it wouldn't work.)
¼ cup honey
1 tablespoon vanilla extract
⅛ teaspoon sea salt
1 cup chopped fruit of choice for topping
Instruction:
Preheat oven to 325 degrees.
Mix all of the dry dough ingredients in a large bowl. Then add in all of the wet dough ingredients. Stir to combine.
Move dough to a silicone baking mat or parchment paper, and roll it out with a rolling pin or something similar. If you need to use your hands, make sure you wet them with water first so that the dough doesn't stick to you.
Using a pastry cutter, cut the dough into 12 equal-sized squares (or rectangles) about 3 (or 2.5) inches wide and 3 inches tall. No need to pull them apart. Once they're done baking, if you can't get them apart easily, just use the pastry cutter again to separate them.
Carefully transfer the baking mat or parchment paper (with the dough on it) to a baking sheet.
Bake for about 10-15 minutes, or until the dough is cooked through and a little bit crispy (like a pie crust would be).
Mix all of the filling ingredients together, except for the fruit.
Once the dough has cooled you can put your layers together. Layer a piece of dough, about 3-4 tablespoons of filling (spread it out), a piece of dough, more filling, a piece of dough, more filling, then some cherries.
Begin a new one. Do this until you run out of dough and filling.

348. Fish Fillet Delux

Ingredients:
4 white fish fillets, about 5 oz each
4 tsp olive oil
Low sodium salt and fresh pepper, to taste
4 sprigs fresh herbs (parsley, rosemary, oregano)
1 lemon, sliced thin
4 large pieces heavy duty aluminum foil,

Instructions:
Place the fish in the center of the foil, season with low sodium salt and pepper and drizzle with olive oil. Place a slice of lemon on top of each piece of fish, then a sprig of herbs on each. Fold up the edges so that it's completely sealed and no steam will escape, creating a loose tent.

Heat half of the grill (on one side) on high heat with the cover closed. When the grill is hot, place the foil packets on the side of the grill with the burners off (indirect heat) and close the grill. Depending on the thickness of your fish, cook 10 to 15 minutes, or until the fish is opaque and cooked through…..serve with green salad and paleo dressing.

349. Roasted Paleo Citrus and Herb Chicken

Ingredients
12 total pieces bone-in chicken thighs and legs
1 medium onion, thinly sliced
1 tbsp dried rosemary
1 tsp dried thyme
1 lemon, sliced thin
1 orange, sliced thin
For the marinade
5 tbsp extra virgin olive oil
6 cloves garlic, minced
1 tbsp honey
Juice of 1 lemon
Juice of 1 orange
1 tbsp Italian seasoning
1 tsp onion powder
Dash of red pepper flakes
Salt and freshly ground pepper, to taste
Instructions
Whisk together all of the marinade ingredients in a small bowl. Place the chicken in a baking dish (or a large Ziploc bag) and pour the marinade over it. Marinate for 3 hours to overnight.
Preheat the oven to 400 degrees F. Place the chicken in a baking dish and arrange with the onion, orange, and lemon slices. Sprinkle with thyme, rosemary, salt and pepper. Cover with aluminum foil and bake for 30 minutes. Remove the foil, baste the chicken, and bake for another 30 minutes uncovered, until the chicken is cooked through.
Notes
Servings: 4-6
Difficulty: Easy

350. Stove-top "Cheesy" Paleo Chicken Casserole

Ingredients

2 cups shredded cooked chicken
1 1/2 cups cooked butternut squash (about 1 small squash)
1/2 cup coconut cream, skimmed from the top of a can of coconut milk
1/4 cup coconut oil, melted
1 heaping cup green peas, thawed
1 tbsp apple cider vinegar
1/2 tsp salt
1/2 tsp oregano
1/2 tsp thyme
1 tbsp fresh parsley, for garnish

Instructions

In a large bowl, mash the butternut squash. Stir in the coconut cream, oil, vinegar, salt, oregano, and thyme. Once everything is combined, add in the shredded chicken and peas.

Place the mixture into a large saucepan and cook over medium heat for 5-8 minutes, until the peas are cooked and squash is creamy. Top with fresh parsley and serve warm.

Notes
Servings: 4-5
Difficulty: Medium

351. Homemade Herbed Paleo Mayonnaise

Ingredients
1 egg (at room temperature)
2 tbsp lemon juice
1 tsp rosemary
1 tsp oregano
½ tsp sea salt
1 cup light olive oil (not EVOO – the flavour will be too strong)
This recipe will make approximately 24 1tbsp servings

Directions
Add egg, lemon juice, rosemary, oregano, and sea salt to a mixing bowl.
Whisk together with an electric mixer on low until well blended. Don't turn off the mixer at any point during this process.
While still whisking, slowly add in your olive oil. Slow is the key word here. Like, one little drizzle at a time slow. Slowly but surely, you'll see the emulsion start to form. Once you see the emulsion forming, continue to add in your olive oil just as slowly until your mayonnaise reaches the desired consistency.
Refrigerate in a glass jar and enjoy! Will last in the fridge approximately one week.

Nutrition Facts Per Serving
Calories: 56
Total Fat: 6.5g
Saturated Fat: 1.0g
Carbs: 0.1g
Protein: 0.2g

352. Homemade Paleo Ketchup with a Kick

Ingredients
1 12 oz can tomato paste
1 cup water
2 tbsp vinegar
½ tsp salt
½ tsp curry powder
½ tsp garlic powder
This recipe makes approximately 32 oz of ketchup, or 64 1tbsp servings.
Directions
Mix all ingredients in a sauce pan and bring to boil on medium-high heat.
Reduce heat to medium-low and simmer while stirring frequently until flavours have blended. (Add more water for thinner ketchup, add less water for thicker)
Transfer to a glass jar and cool before serving.
Nutrition Facts Per Serving
Calories: 5
Total Fat: 0.0g
Sodium: 21mg
Carbs: 1.0g
Protein: 0.7g

353. Homemade Paleo Honey Mustard from Scratch

Ingredients
1/4 cup mustard powder
1/4 cup water
3 tbsp honey
Sea salt, to taste
Instructions
Place the mustard powder and water in a bowl and stir until combined. Add salt and honey to taste. Let stand for at least 15 minutes before serving.
Notes
Servings: about 1/2 cup
Difficulty: Easy

354. All-Natural Homemade Paleo Apple Butter

Ingredients
5 apples, peeled, cored and diced
2/3 cup apple cider
1/3 cup honey
1 tbsp cinnamon
1/2 tsp salt
Pinch of cloves, optional

Instructions
Place all of the ingredients into the slow cooker and stir to evenly coat. Cover and cook on low heat for 6 hours. Let cool slightly and puree in a food processor or blender until smooth.

Notes
Servings: 4-6
Difficulty: Easy

355. Homemade Paleo BBQ Sauce (YUM)

Ingredients
15 oz. organic tomato sauce
1 cup water
1/2 cup apple cider vinegar
1/3 cup honey
1 tbsp lemon juice
2 tsp onion powder
1 1/2 tsp ground black pepper
1 1/2 tsp ground mustard
1 tsp paprika

Instructions
Combine all of the ingredients in a medium saucepan over medium-high heat. Stir to combine. Bring to a boil, and then reduce to simmer for 1 hour. Taste and adjust seasonings as desired. Serve with meat or store in an airtight container in the refrigerator.

Notes
Servings: about 1 1/2 cups
Difficulty: Easy

356. Basil Pesto

Ingredients
1 large bunch of basil (approx. 2 cups)
1/3 cup walnuts or pine nuts
2 medium garlic cloves, minced
1/2 cup Parmigiano Reggiano or other Parmesan cheese (optional)
approx. 1/3 cup extra virgin olive oil
salt and pepper to taste

Instructions
Place basil, nuts, garlic and cheese (optional) in food processor.
Run the food processor, pausing to add olive oil to reach desired consistency.
Salt and pepper to taste.

357. Paleo Chicken Tortilla Soup

Ingredients
2 large chicken breasts, skin removed and cut into ½ inch strips
1 28oz can of diced tomatoes
32 ounces organic chicken broth
1 sweet onion, diced
2 jalepenos, de-seeded and diced
2 cups of shredded carrots
2 cups chopped celery
1 bunch of cilantro chopped fine
4 cloves of garlic, minced - I always use one of these
2 Tbs tomato paste
1 tsp chili powder
1 tsp cumin
sea salt & fresh cracked pepper to taste
olive oil
1-2 cups water

Instructions
In a crockpot or large dutch oven over med-high heat, place a dash of olive oil and about ¼ cup chicken broth. Add onions, garlic, jalapeno, sea salt and pepper and cook until soft, adding more broth as needed.
Then add all of your remaining ingredients and enough water to fill to the top of your pot. Cover and let cook on low for about 2 hrs, adjusting salt & pepper as needed.
Once the chicken is fully cooked, you should be able to shred it very easily. I simply used the back of a wooden spoon and pressed the cooked chicken against the side of the pot. You could also use a fork or tongs to break the chicken apart and into shreds.
Top with avocado slices and fresh cilantro. Enjoy!
This is an easy one-pot meal that's loaded with veggies, low in fat, and full of flavour! You don't need to add cheese or tortilla strips the soup is full of flavour on it's own!

358. Paleo Eggs Benedict on Artichoke Hearts

Eggs Benedict
4 eggs
1 egg white (use from Hollandaise Sauce Recipe below)
250 grams of bacon
4 Artichoke Hearts
3/4 cup of balsamic vinegar
salt and pepper to taste
Hollandaise Sauce
4 egg yolks
1 tbsp of lemon juice
pinch of salt and paprika
¾ cup of melted ghee

Directions

Line a baking sheet with foil and set aside. Preheat your oven to 375 degrees. Deconstruct your artichokes and remove the artichoke hearts. Place the hearts in balsamic vinegar for 20 minutes.

For your Hollandaise Sauce, place a pot of water to simmer on your stove. Melt the ghee in a saucepan. Separate your eggs and place the yolks in a stainless steel cooking bowl. Hold on to the egg whites for the next step.

Remove your hearts from the marinade and place on cookie sheet, brush the tops of them with the egg white and then place your bacon over the artichokes as a second layer. Stick your tray in the oven for 20 minutes.

Back to the sauce, whisk the yolks with the lemon juice and then place your bowl over the simmering water. Slowly add in the ghee and bit of salt and continue to whisk until your sauce doubles in size and is silky. Set aside.

To poach your eggs, turn up the heat on your stove and let the same water get to a rolling boil. Crack your eggs one at a time into a ladle and the slide the egg into the water. Give them about a minute and a half and remove.

Now you are ready to assemble. Grab your artichoke hearts and bacon, then lay your poached egg and pour the Hollandaise silk on top.

359. Hearty Paleo Jambalaya

Ingredients
1 tbsp extra virgin olive oil
8 oz. Andouille sausage, diced
1/2 red bell pepper, diced
1/2 yellow bell pepper, diced
4 cloves garlic, minced
1/2 medium onion, diced
1 14.5-oz. can fire-roasted tomatoes
1 tbsp smoked paprika
1 tsp dried thyme
1 tsp cumin
Dash of cayenne pepper
1 1/2 cups chicken broth
1 large head of cauliflower, coarsely chopped
1 lb. medium shrimp, peeled and deveined
Salt and pepper, to taste
Fresh cilantro, for garnish

Instructions

Heat the olive oil in a Dutch oven or heavy-bottomed saucepan. Add the Andouille sausages and cook for 4-5 minutes until lightly browned. Add the red and yellow peppers, garlic, and onion and stir. Cook for 4 minutes until softened.

Stir in the tomatoes and spices. Pour in the chicken stock and bring to a boil. Once boiling, turn the heat down and simmer for 20 minutes.

Meanwhile, place the cauliflower into a food processor and pulse until it is reduced to the size of rice grains.

Mix in the cauliflower rice to the jambalaya, starting with half of the rice and adding more depending on preference. Simmer for 12-15 minutes until tender. Add the shrimp and cook everything for 5-7 minutes until the shrimp are opaque. Season to taste with salt and pepper. Serve hot, garnished with fresh cilantro.

Notes
Servings: 4-6
Difficulty: Easy

360. Shrimp & Grits (Paleo Style)

For the shrimp
15 pieces raw shrimp, shelled and de-veined
3 tbsp extra virgin olive oil
6 garlic cloves minced, divided
Zest from one lemon
2 tsp dried oregano, divided
2 slices bacon
1/2 large onion, diced
2 tbsp butter
1 tbsp white wine vinegar
1 tsp red pepper flakes
1 tbsp lemon juice
1 tbsp chopped fresh oregano
Salt and freshly ground black pepper, to taste
For the grits
1 large head of cauliflower, cut into florets
1/4 cup almond milk
4 garlic cloves, minced
1 tbsp ghee or butter
1/4 tsp cayenne pepper
Salt and pepper, to taste

Instructions

In a medium bowl mix together the olive oil, 2 cloves of garlic, lemon zest, and 1 teaspoon dried oregano. Place shrimp in the bowl and marinate for 1-3 hours.

Place a couple inches of water in a large pot. Once water is boiling, place steamer insert and then cauliflower florets into the pot and cover. Steam for 12-14 minutes, until completely tender. Drain and return cauliflower to pot.

Add the milk, ghee, and garlic to the cauliflower. Using an immersion blender, combine ingredients. The cauliflower should be fairly thick to resemble the consistency of grits. Season with salt and pepper to taste.

Cook the bacon in a large skillet over medium heat until crispy. Reserving the bacon fat in the pan, set the bacon aside to cool and break into pieces.

Add the butter to the bacon fat in the pan and melt. Add the onion and sauté for 4-5 minutes until softened. Add in the remaining 4 garlic cloves, dried oregano, and the red pepper flakes. Sauté for 1-2 minutes, stirring frequently.

Stir in the white wine vinegar, and then add the shrimp. Cook, stirring frequently, until the shrimp are cooked through, 3-4 minutes. Remove from heat and stir in the lemon juice. Season with salt and pepper. Serve shrimp and onions over grits, with bacon and fresh oregano for garnish.

Notes

Servings: 3-4; Difficulty: Medium

361. How to Make Paleo Cauliflower "Rice"

Ingredients

1 head of cauliflower

½ Vidalia onion

3 cloves of garlic

1 tbsp coconut oil

salt and pepper, to taste

This recipe makes 2-3 servings, depending on the size of your cauliflower.

Instructions

Remove leaves and stem from cauliflower; discard. Grate the entire head of cauliflower until it resembles rice.

Dice the onions and garlic to your desired size.

Add coconut oil to a pan over medium heat. Add in onion and garlic until slightly browned.

Add in grated cauliflower, salt, and pepper and stir until heated.

362. Paleo Cocoa Puffs

Ingredients
¾ Packed Cup of Blanched Almond Flour
1 Cup + 2 Tbsp Tapioca Starch/Flour
½ Cup Cocoa Powder
¼ tsp Salt
⅔ cup Coconut Palm Sugar
2½ tsp. Baking Powder
1 Tbsp Vanilla Extract
⅓ Cup of oil or Melted Butter (dairy or nondairy)
1 Egg + 1 Egg White

Instructions
Preheat Oven to 350 degrees.
Mix together the dry ingredients (Almond Flour, Tapioca Flour, Cocoa Powder, Salt, Palm Sugar, and Baking Powder).
Add in the Vanilla, Oil, and Eggs. Mix really well (don't be afraid to get your hands dirty!)
Line 2 large baking sheets with parchment paper.
Roll teaspoon sized balls of dough (or smaller if you have the patience) in between your palms to create little cocoa puff balls. If you find your hands getting sticky- rinse them off and dry them before continuing and or dust your hands with a little extra tapioca starch.
Use about half the dough to make cocoa puffs for the first baking sheet. Leave a little space between each cocoa puff as they will expand in the oven.
Place the first baking sheet into the oven and bake 18-20 minute. Halfway through baking using a spatula to flip the cocoa puffs over so that the bottoms do not burn.
While the first tray is baking, prepare your second tray of cocoa puffs and follow the same baking instructions.
Let cocoa puffs cool completely before eating. (They will get crispy as they cool).

363. Tantalizing Prawn Skewers

Ingredients:
1 lb jumbo raw tiger prawns, shelled and deveined (weight after peeled)
2 cloves garlic, crushed
Low sodium salt and pepper
8 long wooden skewers

Instructions:
Soak the skewers in water at least 20 minutes to prevent them from burning.

Combine the prawns with crushed garlic and season with low sodium salt and pepper. You can let this marinate for a while, or even overnight.

Heat a clean, lightly oiled grill to medium heat, when the grill is hot add the prawns, careful not to burn the skewers. Grill on both sides for about 6 - 8 minutes total cooking time or until the prawns are opaque and cooked through.

Squeeze lemon juice over the prawns and serve with green salad and my paleo dressing

364. Paleo BLT Frittata

Ingredients
8 eggs
4 slices bacon, cooked and chopped
3-4 cups spinach (or other greens of your choice)
1 large tomato, sliced and seeded
1 tbsp almond milk
1/2 tsp salt
1/4 tsp pepper
2 tbsp chopped fresh basil
1 tbsp extra virgin olive oil

Instructions

Preheat oven to 400 degrees F. In a medium bowl, whisk together the eggs, milk, basil, salt and pepper. Set aside.

Heat olive oil in a 10-inch nonstick skillet over medium heat. Add greens and cook 3-4 minutes until wilted. Add in bacon and stir.

Add egg mixture to the pan and place tomatoes on top. Using a spatula, occasionally lift the edges to allow uncooked egg to run under. When the frittata has set, transfer to the oven and cook for 12-15 minutes or until egg is cooked through. Cut into wedges and serve warm.

Notes
Servings: 5
Difficulty: Easy

365. Extra Easy Broth

Ingredients

4 - 8 lbs of bones, from grass fed animals (depending on the size of stock pot)
2 Tbsp apple cider vinegar
vegetables, carrots, onions, celery
water

Instructions

Roast the bones in the oven at 375 F for 1 hour. This gives a good flavour to the stock.
Remove the bones from the oven and place in a stock pot.
Fill the pot with water - cover the bones.
Add the vegetables - avoid Brussels sprouts, cabbage, broccoli, turnips as these tend to give a bitter flavour to the broth.
Bring the water to a boil and add the vinegar.
Turn the pot down to a simmer.
Allow the broth to simmer for 24 hours or longer.
As it cooks, add water as necessary and skim off any foam.
When finished, strain the broth through a wire mesh and catch the broth in mason jars.
Once cooled, the fat will rise to the top and the broth should gel like gelatine.
The fat can be skimmed off and used for cooking or left in the broth.
The broth will keep refrigerated for 1 week and can also be frozen for months.

Paleo Diet Recipes 365 Days Of Anti-Inflammatory Recipes
By Mercedes Del Rey

About The Author

If you're a sufferer from any kind of immune deficiency disorder, I especially want to extend a warm welcome to you. Welcome, my friend, to my wonderful world of completely safe and natural healing. My name is Mercedes del Rey but my friends and patients call me Merche and I am truly fortunate to live in one of the most beautiful places in the world. My home is in sunny Andalusia in the south of Spain, the place where I was born and where I grew up before travelling to the US to complete my higher education. My life has been blessed in so many ways but, like so many people, I've also had to contend with plenty of problems along the way.

Despite growing up in such a wonderful place, my health has not always been very strong. For example, my immune system was a constant source of worry and I suffered from a series of acute and often debilitating allergies throughout my childhood, sometimes reacting to certain foods and then to the chemicals in ordinary household articles like hand soap and shampoo. I seemed to pick every bug and infection that was going round. A deficient immune system can do that. Eventually, the conditions became severe and I began my long exposure to the medical profession and a cocktail of drugs that were supposed to balance my immune system and calm my allergies but, in the end, they only succeeded in making my life more miserable because of all the unpleasant side effects. Doctors rarely mention the negative consequences of the drugs they prescribe but I could see that my condition was becoming worse rather than getting better.

There were times when I suffered from bouts of depression and a complete lack of confidence, always conscious of the rashes and the embarrassing marks on my skin, the unexplained outbreaks of eczema and the fear of being disfigured by the horrible patches that appeared on my face and body. Sometimes it seemed that my immune system was attacking me rather than protecting me. In some ways, growing up was a nightmare. Like so many other unhappy people, I turned to food as a source of comfort and then I started to gain weight, which made me feel even worse! I was highly strung, super-sensitive, borderline depressed and often miserable. The drugs were no help whatsoever. The fact is that my immune system had been further compromised by the constant stream of allergies and by the medication that had been prescribed for my various conditions. And then, as if out of the blue, I met someone who turned my life around completely.

A friend was very concerned about me. She knew I wasn't sleeping well, that my allergies were a constant source of discomfort and embarrassment, that I was depressed and that I'd hit a low spot in my life where i no longer knew where to turn for help. She recommended someone to me, a very special person, a lady who understood exactly what was wrong with me and who showed me how to change my life forever using the most natural remedies imaginable. Her name is Beran Parry and her knowledge of herbalism opened my life to

Paleo Diet Recipes 365 Days Of Anti-Inflammatory Recipes
By Mercedes Del Rey

an extraordinary world of natural healing. Beran has a very wide knowledge and experience of health, nutrition and all the factors that can contribute to complete wellbeing. The results of her advice and guidance were simply astonishing. My allergies and have disappeared and my immune system is functioning perfectly. I don't even get colds or 'flu anymore, and that in itself is quite remarkable! My mood swings have vanished. I sleep wonderfully and my confidence has soared. I was so impressed by her knowledge and passion for natural healing that I became her pupil and studied with her for several years. She has inspired me to travel the world on my quest to research and investigate herbal medicine and all that it entails.

I visited China, India, Germany, the USA and Canada and met with so many wonderful Naturopathic Doctors and Herbalists along my learning path.

I now practice as a Holistic Nutritionist and I advise my own clients on the use and application of herbal remedies. It was Beran, of course, who encouraged me to write this book and she assisted me with my research and studies. My dearest hope is that it proves to be as useful and helpful to you as her teaching has been to me.

This is not a medical advice book so please always check any remedy with your medical and naturopathic doctor at all times!

May the force of Nature be with you!

Paleo Diet Recipes 365 Days Of Anti-Inflammatory Recipes
By Mercedes Del Rey

DOWNLOAD YOUR FREE PALEO EPIGENETIC DIET EBOOK

AND START LOSING WEIGHT TODAY

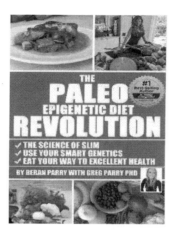

Please search this page over the internet

www.skinnydeliciouslife.com/free-epigenetic-diet-ebook

Paleo Diet Recipes 365 Days Of Anti-Inflammatory Recipes
By Mercedes Del Rey

Before You Go.......

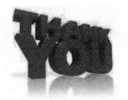

I am so delighted that you have chosen this book and it's been a pleasure writing it for you. My mission is to help as many readers as possible to benefit from the content you have just been reading. So many of us are able to take new information and apply it to our lives with really positive and long lasting consequences and it is my wish that you have been able to take value from the information I have presented.

Thank you for staying with me during this book and for reading it through to the end. I really hope that you have enjoyed the contents and that's why I appreciate your feedback so much. If you could take a couple of minutes to review the book, your views will help me to create more material that you find beneficial.

I am always thrilled to hear from my readers and you can email me personally via the publisher at beranparry@gmail.com if you have any questions about this book or future books. Let us know how we can help you by sending a message to the same email address.

Thanks again for your support and encouragement. I really look forward to reading your review.

Please go to the book product page to complete your review

Stay Healthy!

Paleo Diet Recipes 365 Days Of Anti-Inflammatory Recipes
By Mercedes Del Rey

FOR MORE BY

MERCEDES DEL REY

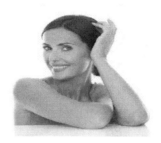

Please search this page over the www.amazon.com

amzn.to/2kSzZnU